High-Yield Internal Medicine

High-Yield Internal Medicine

R. Nirula, M.D.
Resident Physician
Santa Barbara Cottage Hospital
Santa Barbara, California

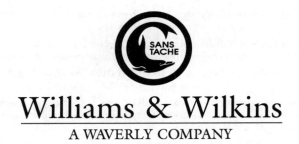

Williams & Wilkins

A WAVERLY COMPANY

BALTIMORE • PHILADELPHIA • LONDON • PARIS • BANGKOK
BUENOS AIRES • HONG KONG • MUNICH • SYDNEY • TOKYO • WROCLAW

Editor: Elizabeth A. Nieginski
Manager, Development Editing: Julie Scardiglia
Managing Editor: Amy G. Dinkel
Marketing Manager: Rebecca Himmelheber
Production Coordinator: Felecia R. Weber
Illustration Planner: Felecia R. Weber
Cover Designer: Karen Klinedinst
Typesetter: Maryland Composition
Printer: Port City Press
Digitized Illustrations: Maryland Composition
Binder: Port City Press

Copyright © 1997 Williams & Wilkins

351 West Camden Street
Baltimore, Maryland 21201-2436 USA

Rose Tree Corporate Center
1400 North Providence Road
Building II, Suite 5025
Media, Pennsylvania 19063-2043 USA

Accurate indications, adverse reactions and dosage schedules for drugs are provided in this book, but it is possible that they may change. The reader is urged to review the package information data of the manufacturers of the medications mentioned.

Printed in the United States of America

First Edition

Library of Congress Cataloging-in-Publication Data

Nirula, R. (Raminder)
   High-yield internal medicine / R. Nirula. — 1st ed.
     p. cm.
   Includes index.
   ISBN 0-683-18044-4
   1. Internal medicine—Outlines, syllabi, etc. I. Title.
   [DNLM: 1. Internal Medicine—outlines. WB 18.2 N721h 1997]
RC59.N55 1997
616—dc21
DNLM/DLC
for Library of Congress   97-7043
                                        CIP

The publishers have made every effort to trace the copyright holders for borrowed material. If they have inadvertently overlooked any, they will be pleased to make the necessary arrangements at the first opportunity.

To purchase additional copies of this book, call our customer service department at **(800) 638-0672** or fax orders to **(800) 447-8438**. For other book services, including chapter reprints and large quantity sales, ask for the Special Sales department.

Canadian customers should call **(800) 665-1148**, or fax **(800) 665-0103**. For all other calls originating outside of the United States, please call **(410) 528-4223** or fax us at **(410) 528-8550**.

Visit Williams & Wilkins on the Internet: http://www.wwilkins.com or contact our customer service department at **custserv@wwilkins.com**. Williams & Wilkins customer service representatives are available from 8:30 am to 6:00 pm. EST, Monday through Friday, for telephone access.

97 98 99 00
1 2 3 4 5 6 7 8 9 10

Dedication

For my patient and beautiful wife, Julie,
and our endless source of joy, Kieran.

Derek and I anxiously awaited the emergence of our housemate from his slumber. The door opened, and a sunken shadow appeared in the doorway. Just one more step . . . that's it. Then it happened. The silence was finally broken and our hopes were vindicated. The sounds of water hitting the flat surface of a squarish head echoed throughout the house. Then a split second of silence swallowed the walls, only to be smashed by the shrill of obscenities and the boyish laughter of two grown men.

I turned to Derek with a devilish look, realizing finally the true gift of gravity
and the laws of physics.

For Sir Isaac Newton

Contents

Preface xi

1 Rheumatic Diseases 1

    I. Osteoarthritis and Rheumatoid Arthritis   1
    II. Crystal-related Joint Diseases   4
    III. Spondyloarthropathies   7
    IV. Systemic Lupus Erythematosus (SLE)   11
    V. Systemic Sclerosis (Scleroderma)   12
    VI. Polymyositis and Dermatomyositis   14
    VII. Sjögren's Disease   14
    VIII. Vasculitic Syndromes   15

2 Endocrinologic and Metabolic Disorders 20

    I. Disorders of the Pituitary Gland   20
    II. Disorders of the Thyroid Gland   24
    III. Disorders of the Parathyroid Gland   28
    IV. Glucose Homeostasis   31
    V. Adrenal Gland Dysfunction   34
    VI. Female Reproductive Disorders   38
    VII. Male Reproductive Disorders   42
    VIII. Disorders of Bone Metabolism   43

3 Renal, Fluid, and Electrolyte Disorders 46

    I. Renal Failure   46
    II. Abnormal Urinalysis and Glomerulonephropathy   48
    III. Renal Calculi   50
    IV. Renovascular Disease   51
    V. Assessment and Diagnosis of Volume and Electrolyte Disorders   52

4 Cardiovascular Diseases 60

    I. Congestive Heart Failure (CHF)   60
    II. Ischemic Heart Disease (IHD)   62
    III. Valvular Heart Disease   63
    IV. Cardiomyopathies and Pericardial Disease   67
    V. Deep Venous Thrombosis, Pulmonary Embolus, and Aortic Aneurysms   71
    VI. Systemic Hypertension   74

5   Pulmonary Diseases   77

    I.   Obstructive Lung Disease   77
    II. Diffuse Interstitial Lung Disease   82
   III. Adult Respiratory Distress Syndrome (ARDS)   85
   IV. Disorders of the Pleural Space, Mediastinum, and Chest Wall   86
    V. Neoplasms of the Lung   90
   VI. Pulmonary Disease of Unknown Etiology   94

6   Gastrointestinal Disorders   96

    I.   Diseases of the Esophagus and Stomach   96
    II. Diseases of the Small Intestine   101
   III. Diseases of the Colon, Rectum, and Anus   109
   IV. Pancreatic Disorders   116
    V. Biliary Tract Disease   118
   VI. Liver Diseases   119

7   Neurologic Diseases   124

    I.   Cerebrovascular Disease   124
    II. Disorders of Higher Cognitive Function   127
   III. Dementia   129
   IV. Seizure Disorders   130
    V. Headaches   132
   VI. Movement Disorders   134
  VII. Spinal Cord Syndromes   137
 VIII. Neurocutaneous Syndromes   141
   IX. Peripheral Neural Disorders   142
    X. Neuromuscular Disorders   145
   XI. Multiple Sclerosis (MS)   148

8   Oncologic Diseases   150

    I.   Head and Neck Carcinoma   150
    II. Renal and Bladder Carcinoma   150
   III. Prostatic Carcinoma   151
   IV. Gastric Carcinoma   152
    V. Pancreatic Carcinoma   153
   VI. Colorectal Carcinoma   154
  VII. Lung Carcinoma   156
 VIII. Multiple Myeloma   158
   IX. The Lymphomas   159
    X. The Leukemias   160

9   Hematologic Diseases   164

    I.   Anemias   164
    II. Hematocrit Disorders   173
   III. Leukocyte Disorders   174
   IV. Hemostasis and Coagulation Disorders   177

10   Infectious Diseases **182**

   I.   Central Nervous System (CNS) Infections   182
   II.   Head and Neck Infections   184
   III.   Respiratory Tract Infections   184
   IV.   Gastrointestinal Infections   190
   V.   Genital and Sexually Transmitted Diseases   190
   VI.   Urinary Tract Infections (UTIs)   192
   VII.   Osteomyelitis and Joint Infections   193
   VIII.   Other Infectious Syndromes   194

lyme disease : New York, NJ, Connecticut, Rhode Island,
Massachusetts, Pennsylvania, Wisconsin, Minnesota)
erythema migrans 80% pt has,

-prevent B. burgdorferi : DEET application prior to
hunting   Ixodes ricinus
         (N,N,-diethyl-m-toluamide)
                    DEET.

Preface

Upon completing my clerkship in Internal Medicine, I must admit that I believed I had reached a new level in my training. My senior residents had congratulated me and patted me on the back, telling me how my knowledge base was "phenomenal" and my diagnostic skills "superb." Having my ego boosted was a wonderful sensation, and so I looked forward to the following week with vigorous delight, when I would have the opportunity to review my evaluation. The evaluation was completed by the Chief-of-Staff of Internal Medicine—a somewhat rust-colored individual with a tired look that seemed to say, "Only two more years until retirement!" Needless to say, I had never worked with him and was content with this fact. Still, I was confident that the praise which I had received from my upper colleagues had traversed the compounded cerumen of his external ear. As I flipped through my evaluations, I triumphantly reached the Internal Medicine section. With the excitement of a child on Christmas morning, I read, ". . . Dr. Nirula's performance has been fully satisfactory . . . ."

"What?!" I checked the sheet to ensure that this was, in fact, the appropriately filed evaluation. *Fully satisfactory?* What does *that* mean? Is that somehow better than *simply satisfactory*, and can someone be *partially satisfactory*, or *barely satisfactory*? Either you are satisfactory or you are not. Who was this guy trying to kid?

Reeling from my less than gratifying review, I rationalized my meager evaluation as being the writings of an eccentric and *fully psychotic* individual. This rationalization allowed me to cope with the remainder of my training with minimal emotional trauma.

While the experience left me jaded, I still firmly believe that clinicians should attempt to learn as much as possible during their training. Time constraints are incredible during this phase, and so reading should be devoted to sources that are concise, informative, and pertinent to one's education. *High-Yield Internal Medicine* is such a book. It gives useful information about common medical illnesses, presented in such a way that a young clinician can develop a rational approach to clinical medicine. In my humble opinion, it is more than a *fully satisfactory* resource.

R. Nirula, M.D.

Rheumatoid arthritis affects the MCPs and spares the DIPs.

1

Rheumatic Diseases

I. OSTEOARTHRITIS AND RHEUMATOID ARTHRITIS

A. Osteoarthritis (OA) *path p346*

1. **General characteristics**
   a. OA is the **most common rheumatic disease.**
   b. **Incidence** increases with **age, wear and tear,** and **obesity.**
   c. OA is characterized by **degeneration of cartilage,** with reactive changes and new bone formation that leads to **bony spurs; subchondral cysts** may also form in the juxta-articular bone.
   d. OA may be classified as **primary OA or secondary OA,** depending on the presence or absence of an underlying etiologic factor.
   e. Some **causes for secondary OA** include **previous trauma to the involved joint, congenital hip dysplasia, avascular necrosis** of the capital femoral epiphysis, **post inflammatory disorders** (rheumatoid or infective arthritis), **metabolic disorders** (calcium pyrophosphate deposition disorder, Wilson's disease, hemochromatosis).

2. **Clinical features**

   sparing the MCPs

   a. **Symptoms** include gradual onset of **deep pain** that worsens with activity and is relieved by rest; **morning stiffness** that lasts < 30 minutes; and **painful range of motion.**
   b. **Signs and symptoms** of late-stage OA include **tenderness, crepitus,** and **joint deformity.**
   c. In the **hand, Heberden's nodes** (enlarged distal interphalangeal [DIP] joints) and **Bouchard's nodes** (enlarged proximal interphalangeal [PIP] joints) may form.
   d. In the **knee,** a disproportionate **loss of cartilage from medial or lateral compartments** may give rise to **genu valgus** or **varus.**
   e. In the **hip, pain** occurs in the **groin, inner thigh, knee** or **buttocks,** and **internal rotation and extension are lost.**
   f. In the **foot,** the **first metatarsophalangeal joint** is commonly affected.
   g. In the **spine,** the **L3–4 intervertebral disc** is commonly affected, and **cauda equina syndrome with sphincter dysfunction** may occur.

3. **Differential diagnosis** includes seronegative rheumatoid arthritis; psoriatic arthritis or Reiter's syndrome; chronic infective arthritis; and tendonitis and/or bursitis.

4. **Laboratory findings**

1

ESR normal

a. Results of **hematologic studies** are **usually normal,** including the erythrocyte sedimentation rate (ESR).

b. **Synovial fluid aspiration** indicates **mild inflammation** (<2000 cells per mm^3, <30% neutrophils); **no crystals;** and **good mucin clot formation** (unlike inflammatory aspirates). *asymmetric narrowing*

c. **Radiography** indicates **joint space narrowing, marginal osteophytes,** and **subchondral cysts;** erosions are usually *not* present.

5. Treatment

a. Joint preservation can be achieved through **weight reduction, physical therapy,** and **mechanical devices** (canes, braces).

initial Rx b. **Acetaminophen,** aspirin, and other nonsteroidal anti-inflammatory drugs **(NSAIDs)** are **beneficial.**

c. **Systemic corticosteroids** are **contraindicated,** and **intra-articular steroid injections** should be used for **acute flare-ups** only.

d. In **severely affected joints, surgery** to correct severe deformity or complete joint replacement may be indicated.

B. **Rheumatoid arthritis (RA)**

1. General characteristics

a. **RA** is a **chronic, systemic, inflammatory disorder** more commonly begins in women during their childbearing years.

b. RA involves an **inflammation and hypertrophy of the synovium,** with infiltration by lymphocytes; the resulting **immune complex formation leads to an immune reaction.**

c. The **inflammatory process** eventually **leads to ulcerations** in the cartilage, surrounding ligaments, and bone.

2. Clinical features

a. **Symptoms** include **fatigue, malaise,** and **generalized musculoskeletal pain** over weeks to months, **followed by specific joint pain, tenderness, redness, and swelling.**

b. **Symmetric joints** of the hands, wrists, elbows, shoulders, and feet are **frequently affected.** Patients may initially be seen with **prolonged morning** *>30 min* **stiffness,** with symptoms being **aggravated by movement.**

spares DIP c. In the **hand, metacarpophalangeal (MCP) joints** and **PIPs** are affected; **DIPs** are not affected (unlike OA); **ulnar deviation of fingers** and **palmar subluxation of the PIPs** are common; **swan-neck deformities** (hyperextension of PIP and flexion of DIP) or **boutonniere deformities** (flexion of PIP and extension of DIP) occur later in the disease process.

d. In the **wrists, decreased dorsiflexion, carpal tunnel syndrome,** and **atrophy of the thenar eminence** occur.

e. In the **elbows, flexion contractures** tend to occur early in the disease process.

f. In the **neck, pain and stiffness** associated with **cervical vertebral erosion** may progress to **atlantoaxial subluxation.**

g. In the **knee, patellar tap** reveals effusion, which may yield to a Baker's cyst.

h. In the **feet, cocking up of toes** and **subluxation of metatarsal heads** result in a **clawlike appearance.** *nodules*

i. **Subcutaneous nodules** at the elbows, **occiput,** and **sacrum** develop in 20% to 25% of patients and are associated with **seropositive disease.**

j. Clinical course

   (1) **Sporadic course** with periods of remission has a **favorable prognosis.**

   (2) **Insidious progression** with periodic debilitating flare-ups as well as joint subluxation and joint contractures with fibrosis has a **variable prognosis.**

(3) **"Malignant" rapid progressive deterioration** is characterized by systemic symptoms of weight loss, synovitis, rheumatoid nodules, high levels of rheumatoid factor, vasculitis, scleritis, pulmonary nodules, neuropathy, and myopericarditis.

3. **Differential diagnosis**

a. **Systemic lupus erythematosus** often involves joints symmetrically but is usually not deforming.

b. **Spondyloarthropathies** are distinguished from RA by their **sacroiliac and axial spine involvement.**

c. **Systemic sclerosis** is characterized by **short-lived joint inflammation** and characteristic **skin changes.**

d. **Rheumatic fever,** uncommon in adults, should be considered if an associated pharyngitis and migratory arthritis are present.

e. **Polymyalgia rheumatica** is distinguished from RA by intermittent, non-deforming arthritis.

f. **Lyme disease** is difficult to distinguish from RA without the history of a tick bite and characteristic skin, cardiac, or central nervous system (CNS) changes.

4. **Laboratory findings**

a. **Hematologic studies** indicate normochromic-normocytic or hypochromic-microcytic anemia, thrombocytosis (500 to 700 × 10^9/L), and elevated ESR; positive results for rheumatoid factor are useful but not diagnostic.

b. **Synovial fluid aspiration** reveals 5000 to 40,000 cells/mm^3 with 50% to 70% polymorphonuclear neutrophils(PMNs), decreased complement, and poor mucin clot formation.

c. **Radiography** indicates evidence of joint deformities as described previously as well as the presence of cysts, loss of cartilage, and erosive changes (Figure 1-1).

5. **Treatment**

a. **First-line treatment** involves education, rest, exercise, and relief of joint pain and inflammation with NSAIDs.

b. A **6-month trial** of **hydroxychloroquine** (antimalarial) or **gold** may be necessary for unremitting disease, followed by penicillamine, methotrexate, or azathioprine if the hydroxychloroquine trial is unsuccessful.

c. **Intra-articular corticosteroids** may be beneficial for treating flare-ups.

d. **Orthopedic surgery** may be beneficial for impending or severe joint deformities.

e. **Medications** used to treat RA may cause **side effects.**

(1) **Salicylates** may cause gastrointestinal (GI) ulcers, hearing loss and other CNS side effects, platelet function inhibition, and liver function test abnormalities.

(2) **Gold** may cause pruritic skin rash, mouth ulcers, and transient leukopenia.

(3) **Penicillamine** may cause thrombocytopenia, leukopenia, nephrotic syndrome, GI upset, obliterative bronchitis, and alterations in taste perceptions.

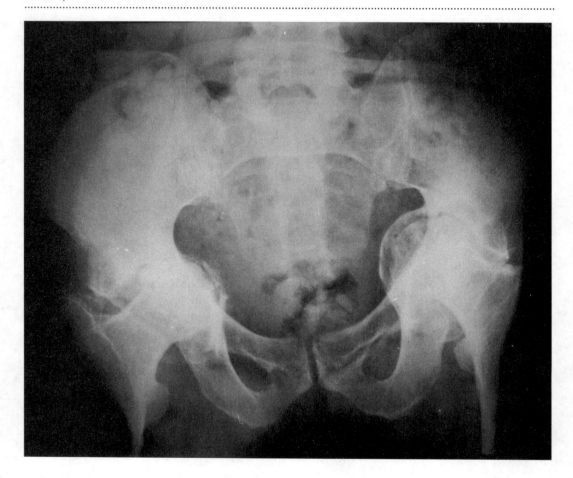

Figure 1-1.   A patient with rheumatoid arthritis who has marked protrusion of the acetabula and joint space narrowing. A hallmark of this disease is symmetric joint involvement.

II. CRYSTAL-RELATED JOINT DISEASES

A. Gout

1. General characteristics
   a. Gout occurs **secondary to a disorder of purine metabolism** that leads to hyperuricemia and, hence, intra-articular and extra-articular urate deposition.
   b. Gout commonly affects **middle-aged men.**
   c. **Ninety percent** of gout patients are **underexcreters of uric acid** (< 700 mg/dl) usually as a result of renal disease secondary to volume depleted states (e.g., adrenal insufficiency, diabetes insipidus); drugs such as acetylsalicylic acid (ASA), which decrease uric acid excretion; or organic acid accumulation (e.g., ketones, lactic acid, which compete with uric acid for renal excretion).
   d. **Ten percent** of gout patients are overproducers of uric acid who excrete >750 mg/dl on a normal diet due to a purine metabolic enzyme deficiency

no ASA for gout ∴ ↓ uric acid excretion

10%

or secondary to increased nucleic acid turnover (e.g., myeloproliferative disorders, psoriasis, chemotherapy).

2. Clinical features

    a. There are **two clinical stages** of gout:

        (1) In **asymptomatic hyperuricemia,** urate deposition is absent, but increased serum uric acid concentration puts the patient at risk for acute gouty arthritis.

        (2) In **acute** gouty arthritis, lower extremity, monoarticular arthritis (50% of cases affect first metatarsophalangeal joint) produces sudden tenderness, erythema, warmth, and swelling that resolves in a few days.

    b. A **mild fever** may be present in the acute phase.

    c. Attacks may be **triggered by trauma, alcohol, stress,** or **acute medical illness.**

    d. **Chronic tophaceous gout** develops in advanced cases where urate crystals deposit within the subcutaneous tissues, which can therefore be **mistaken for the rheumatoid nodules of RA.**

    e. A **common complication** of gout is **acute obstructive uropathy** leading to acute renal failure.

3. **Differential diagnosis** includes septic arthritis; other crystal deposition diseases; and rheumatoid arthritis, especially in the presence of gouty tophi, which can be mistaken for rheumatoid nodules.

4. Laboratory findings

    a. **Hematologic studies** indicate mild leukocytosis and a mildly elevated ESR.

    b. **Elevated serum uric acid levels** are helpful but not diagnostic, because more than 10% of patients have normal serum uric acid levels during an acute attack.

    c. **Synovial fluid aspiration** indicates the presence of monosodium urate crystals (needle-shaped and negatively birefringent in polarized light) in the synovial fluid; cell count is 10,000 to 60,000 cells/mm^3 ($>$ 70% PMNs).

    d. **Aspiration of gouty tophi** reveals urate crystals, which differentiate the gouty tophi from rheumatoid nodules.

    e. **Radiography** is usually of little value during the acute attack, because radiographs reveal only soft-tissue swelling.

        (1) However, radiography may **help exclude septic arthritis** from the differential diagnosis, because gout is characteristically accompanied by destructive changes.

        (2) In the case of **chronic tophaceous gout,** radiographs may show punched-out erosions in the subchondral bone.

5. Treatment

    a. **NSAIDs** such as indomethacin are effective in relieving the pain of an acute attack.

    b. **Colchicine** may be used early in the acute attack, especially if the patient has a history of gastric ulcer or conditions associated with decreased renal perfusion (contraindications for the use of NSAIDs).

    c. **Intra-articular corticosteroids** may be effective treatment if the aforementioned therapies are poorly tolerated or if the patient has severe monoarticular disease.

    d. **Uric acid–lowering agents** should not be used during the acute attack phase because they can prolong the duration of the attack.

    e. **Acetylsalicylic acid** should not be given for relief of pain during the acute attack because it interferes with uric acid excretion.

decrease uric acid excretion

    f. **Prophylaxis of attacks** can be achieved with daily **low-dose colchicine or NSAIDs.**

    g. Patients who have **persistent gout, visible tophi, or recurrent uric acid renal calculi** should be treated with uric acid–lowering agents after the acute phase.

    h. **Uricosuric drugs,** such as probenecid and sulfinpyrazone, lower uric acid levels by decreasing tubular uric acid reabsorption; this effect is blocked by ASA.

    i. **Allopurinol** is a xanthine oxidase inhibitor (xanthine oxidase is an enzyme that converts hypoxanthine and xanthine to uric acid) and therefore lowers serum uric acid levels.

        (1) This drug is appropriate for patients with a history of uric acid renal calculi (contraindication to the use of uricosuric agents), or patients with decreased renal function who would therefore gain little benefit from uricosuric agents.

        (2) **Allopurinol toxicity** is characterized by fever, leukocytosis, decreased renal function, and pruritic rash, which may occur in up to 5% of treated patients; therefore, allopurinol should be used only if uricosuric agents are contraindicated or are likely to be ineffective.

B. **Calcium pyrophosphate dihydrate deposition disease (CPPD)**

  1. **General characteristics**

    a. CPPD is also known as **pseudogout.**

    b. CPPD may be **hereditary** (autosomal dominant), idiopathic, or associated with other metabolic disorders (e.g., hemochromatosis and hyperparathy- _—(AP)_ roidism). _hypothyroidism , amyloidosis , hemochromatosis_

  2. **Clinical features** _(↑SH)_   _(transferrin saturation)_

    a. **Attacks** are common after surgery, trauma, or medical illness.

    b. **Acute onset of warmth, erythema, swelling,** and **tenderness** occurs most commonly in the knee as well as in the first metatarsophalangeal joint.

    c. Attacks last for a few days and are self-limited.

    d. Signs and symptoms may spread to adjacent joints.

    e. **Fever** and **leukocytosis** may also be present.

    f. **CPPD crystals** may be found in synovial fluid, tendons, ligaments, and cartilage.

  3. **Differential diagnosis** includes septic arthritis, gout, and OA.

  4. **Laboratory findings**

    a. **Synovial fluid aspiration** reveals rhomboid crystals that demonstrate weakly positive results for birefringence in polarized light.

    b. **Radiography** indicates punctate and linear densities in the articular hyaline cartilage.

chondrocalcinosis

        (1) **Calcific deposits** may be seen in tendons, ligaments, and articular cartilage.

        (2) **Hooklike osteophytes** and **subchondral cysts** are not uncommon.

        (3) Although these changes can suggest OA, their **presence in joints** such as the wrist, elbow, and shoulder (where OA is uncommon) **suggests CPPD.**

  5. **Treatment**

    a. Repeated **aspiration of synovial fluid** can shorten the duration of attacks.

    b. **NSAIDs** and **intra-articular corticosteroids** are useful in alleviating painful symptoms.

    c. An effective therapy to remove CPPD crystals is currently unavailable.

colchicine 0.6 mg Bid reduce the fequency of pseudogout attacks.

newly diagnosed CPPD need following study (1) TSH for hypothyroidism (2) Ca++, phos, Magnesium, transferrin saturation for hemochromatosis (3) alkaline phosphatase for hyperparathyroidism

C. Hemochromatosis

    1. General characteristics

        a. Hemochromatosis is an **inherited disorder of iron metabolism** associated with excessive body iron stores.

        b. Hemochromatosis may occur secondary to **repeated blood transfusions.**

        c. Hemosiderin accumulates in the synovial lining and articular cartilage.

    2. Clinical features

        a. Hemochromatosis primarily affects the **second and third MCP joints.**

        b. Other joints may secondarily become affected in association with CPPD deposition.

    3. Laboratory findings

        a. **Serum analysis** indicates elevated serum iron and ferritin levels.

        b. **Synovial fluid aspiration** indicates < 1000 cells/mm^3, good mucin clot formation, and iron levels that reflect those of serum.

        c. **Radiography** reveals chondrocalcinosis in 50% of cases.

    4. Treatment

        a. **Phlebotomy** to decrease body iron stores does not seem to affect already established arthropathy.

        b. **NSAIDs** may provide symptomatic relief.

III. SPONDYLOARTHROPATHIES

A. General characteristics

    1. Spondyloarthropathies are a **group of inflammatory arthritides** that are distinct from RA and are therefore seronegative.

    2. They are distinguished from RA by predominant, asymmetric involvement of the axial skeleton and the sacroiliac joints.

    3. Types of spondyloarthropathies discussed here include ankylosing spondylitis, Reiter's syndrome, psoriatic arthritis, and enteropathic arthropathies.

B. Ankylosing spondylitis

    1. General characteristics

        a. Ankylosing spondylitis primarily involves the sacroiliac joints and spine.

        b. HLA-B27 is associated with ankylosing spondylitis; therefore, a positive family history is often present.

        c. Onset usually occurs in the second and third decades of life.

    2. Clinical features

        a. **Symptoms** include fatigue, weight loss, low-grade fever, insidious onset of lower back discomfort that persists for several months, and morning stiffness that improves with exercise and worsens with rest.

        b. Patients experience decreased spinal mobility, loss of lumbar lordosis, and increased thoracic kyphosis.

        c. **Peripheral joint involvement** and **pulmonary fibrosis** are features of **severe disease.**

        d. **Transient uveitis** (pain, redness, and photophobia) develops in up to 25% of patients.

    3. Differential diagnosis

        a. **Mechanical low backache** usually **worsens** with activity and is **relieved** by rest.

    b. Other spondyloarthropathies can be distinguished from ankylosing spondylitis on the basis of associated symptoms described later in this chapter.

  4. **Laboratory findings**
    a. **HLA-B27 testing,** although highly suggestive of the diagnosis, is costly and should not be performed unless the diagnosis is uncertain.
    b. **Radiography** indicates squaring of the superior and inferior margins of the vertebral bodies, which leads to **"bamboo" spine** (Figure 1-2); destruction of cartilage and subchondral erosions give the appearance of widened sacroiliac joints.

  5. **Treatment**
    a. **Physical therapy** is critical to preserve function and prevent further deformity.
    b. **NSAIDs** provide relief of pain so that patients can achieve maximum function.
    c. Due to thoracic deformities and the risk of fibrosis, **smoking** is **severely discouraged** in this population.

C. **Reiter's syndrome**
  1. **General characteristics**
    a. Reiter's syndrome is also known as **reactive arthritis.**
    b. Reiter's syndrome occurs secondary to chlamydial urethritis or gastrointestinal infections by *Shigella, Salmonella, Yersinia,* and *Campylobacter.*
    c. Because organisms are not cultured from arthritic joints, Reiter's syndrome is a reactive arthritis.
    d. The disease often occurs in **young adulthood.**

  2. **Clinical features**
    a. Signs and symptoms of Reiter's syndrome usually occur 2 to 4 weeks after the initial infection.
    b. Acute onset is characterized by asymmetric arthritis in knees and ankles.
    c. Three typical features include:
      (1) **Diffuse swelling of finger(s) or toe(s)** which gives rise to the "sausage digit."
      (2) **Tenderness** of the **Achilles tendon insertion.**
      (3) **Low back pain** associated with sacroiliitis.
    d. Forty percent of patients develop mild, noninfectious, transient **conjunctivitis** and 3% to 5% develop disabling iritis, uveitis, or corneal ulceration.
    e. **Mucocutaneous lesions** include balanitis circinata (small, shallow, painless ulcers of the glans penis) and keratoderma blennorrhagicum (hyperkeratotic scaling skin lesions similar to psoriasis) on the palms and soles.
    f. The majority of patients experience recurrent episodes of **arthritis,** but severe disability is rare.

  3. **Laboratory findings**
    a. **Hematologic studies** indicate elevated ESR and leukocytosis.
    b. **Reiter's syndrome** is HLA-B27–linked.
    c. **Synovial fluid aspiration** indicates 500 to 75,000 cells/mm^3 with a predominance of PMNs.
    d. **Radiography** reveals erosions and periosteal changes at the ischial tuberosities, greater trochanter, and Achilles tendon insertion.
      (1) Radiography also reveals **sacroiliitis.**
      (2) **Asymmetric syndesmophytes** are found along the spine (unlike ankylosing spondylitis, in which they are symmetric and contiguous).

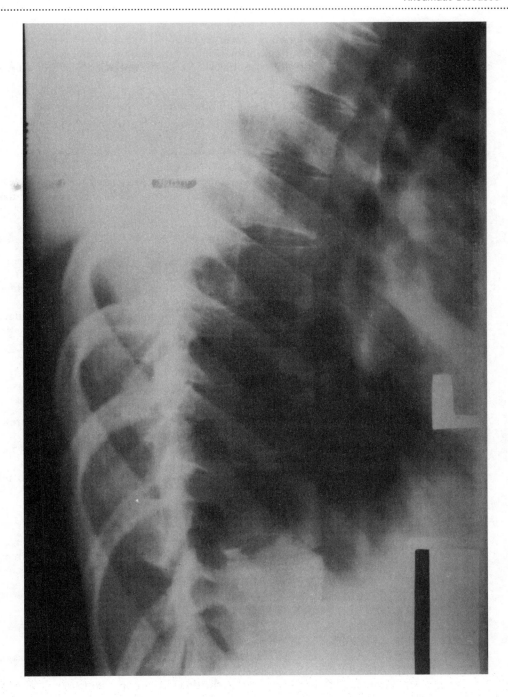

Figure 1-2.   Radiograph showing a characteristic feature of ankylosing spondylitis, that is, squaring of the anterior surface of the vertebrae in the thoracolumbar region (the so-called bamboo spine).

4. Treatment
   a. **NSAIDs** are the primary line of therapy.
   b. No evidence exists that antibiotics alter the disease course.
   c. **Systemic corticosteroids** are ineffective, but **intra-articular steroids** for severe monoarthritic disease produce relief.
   d. **Topical corticosteroids** may be prescribed for keratoderma blennorrhagicum and conjunctivitis.
   e. **Sulfasalazine** is the second line of therapy if NSAIDs are inadequate.

D. Psoriatic arthritis

1. **General characteristics**
   a. Psoriatic arthritis is an inflammatory arthritis **associated with psoriasis.**
   b. Approximately 7% of patients who have psoriasis have some form of inflammatory arthritis.
   c. Several HLA types have been associated with this form of arthritis.

2. **Clinical features**
   a. **Disease onset** occurs in the **30s and 40s,** with skin lesions followed by arthritis.
   b. The majority of patients have **peripheral, asymmetric joint involvement;** spinal involvement is not uncommon.
   c. Approximately 25% of patients have a **symmetric polyarthritis** similar to that of RA.
   d. Patients may develop **sausage digits** as in Reiter's syndrome.
   e. **Psoriatic lesions** are commonly found on the extensor surfaces.
   f. **Nail involvement** may include pitting and longitudinal ridges.
   g. **Conjunctivitis or anterior uveitis** may occur in up to 30% of patients.

3. **Laboratory findings**
   a. **Serum analysis** reveals mildly elevated ESR; hyperuricemia may be present with cases of severe psoriasis.
   b. **Synovial fluid aspiration** reveals mild inflammation, with 2000 to 15,000 cells/mm^3 and a predominance of PMNs.
   c. **Radiography** indicates distal interphalangeal erosions progressing to telescoping joints.
      (1) Asymmetric sacroiliitis progressing to fusion is also common.
      (2) Isolated axial syndesmophytes may be seen at any level.

4. Treatment
   a. **NSAIDs** such as indomethacin are effective in relieving joint symptoms.
   b. Severe disease may require **intra-articular corticosteroid** treatment.
   c. **Methotrexate, penicillamine, gold,** and **hydroxychloroquine** are effective second-line agents.

E. Enteropathic arthropathies

1. **Clinical features**
   a. Enteropathic arthropathies are forms of **polyarticular arthritis** and are associated with ulcerative colitis or Crohn's disease.
   b. **Peripheral (lower extremity) arthritis** exists in approximately 20% of patients, whereas sacroiliitis predominates in another 20%.
   c. **HLA-B27** is not linked with lower extremity arthritic syndrome, but HLA-B27 linkage is present in the sacroiliitis form.
   d. **Peripheral arthritis** tends to exacerbate with flare-ups of the bowel disease, whereas the **sacroiliitis** tends to progress independent of the bowel disease.

   2. Laboratory findings
      a. **Synovial fluid aspiration** reveals effusions that are mildly to severely inflammatory and nonspecific.
      b. **Radiography** indicates that:
         (1) Sacroiliitis is symmetric, as in ankylosing spondylitis.
         (2) No destructive changes are present in the peripheral arthritis form.

   3. Treatment
      a. Successful management of the inflammatory bowel disease alleviates the peripheral arthritis.
      b. Therapy for the sacroiliitis form is identical to that for ankylosing spondylitis.

IV. SYSTEMIC LUPUS ERYTHEMATOSUS (SLE)

A. General characteristics

   1. SLE is **most common in women during their reproductive years, especially in blacks.**

   2. SLE is an **acute and chronic inflammatory process** with multiple organ involvement. The disease is linked to both HLA-DR2 and HLA-DR3.

   3. SLE is believed to occur **secondary to increased lymphocyte activity,** which leads to formation of autoantibodies → immune complex deposition → tissue damage → fibrinoid necrosis.

   4. A variety of symptoms may be present at any one time, and symptoms may develop over months to years.

   5. SLE may be **drug-induced** (e.g., hydralazine, procainamide).

B. Clinical features

   1. Common **constitutional symptoms** include fatigue, weight loss, and fever.

   2. **Skin** signs and symptoms include facial butterfly rash, alopecia, and photosensitivity.

   3. **Nervous system** signs and symptoms include personality disorders, seizures, psychoses, and mononeuritis multiplex.

   4. **Cardiac** signs and symptoms include pericardial effusions and myocarditis.

   5. **Pulmonary** signs and symptoms include pleuritis, pleural effusions, pneumonitis.

   6. Common **GI tract** signs and symptoms include nonspecific abdominal complaints; less common signs and symptoms include infarction, perforation, and hemorrhage occurring secondary to bowel vasculitis.

   7. **Renal** signs include any type of glomerulonephropathy.

   8. Common **musculoskeletal** signs include symmetrical peripheral arthralgias (which are easily confused with RA); damage is limited to tendons and ligaments, with relatively no articular deformities.

   9. A common **reticuloendothelial** sign is hepatosplenomegaly with lymphadenopathy; some patients develop functional hyposplenism, which results in increased risk of bacterial infection.

  10. **Vasculitic** complications include purpuric lesions (which may progress to necrosis) on fingertips, toes, and extensor surfaces.

C. **Differential diagnosis** includes RA, mixed connective tissue diseases, vasculitic syndromes (see VIII), and drug-induced SLE.

D. **Laboratory findings**

   1. **Hematologic studies** reveal anemia characteristic of chronic disease (normochromic-normocytic) or Coombs' positive hemolytic anemia; lymphopenia secondary to autoantibodies (more common than leukopenia); thrombocytopenia; elongated thromboplastin time (not corrected by addition of normal plasma to serum because clotting factors are inhibited by autoantibodies).

   2. **Serum analysis** reveals positive results for the presence of antinuclear antibodies (ANA); this test is the standard screening test for SLE, but is not specific for the disease.

   a. **Antibodies to double-stranded DNA (Anti-dsDNA) and a small nuclear ribonucleoprotein (Anti-Sm)** are specific to SLE.

   b. **ANAs to histones** suggest the drug-induced form of SLE.

   c. **Hypocomplementemia** (C3 and C4) is highly suggestive of the diagnosis.

   d. **False-positive** Venereal Disease Research Laboratories test **(for syphilis)** may occur.

E. **Treatment**

   1. Patients should receive **education** to cope with a chronic illness.

   2. **NSAIDs,** in anti-inflammatory doses, are a useful treatment for serositis, fever, and joint pain. *[handwritten: COX2-inh]*

   3. **Corticosteroids** are used topically for treating cutaneous manifestations and systemically for treating multiple organ involvement and result in a generally good response.

   4. **Hydroxychloroquine or chloroquine** has been used for cutaneous manifestations and milder forms of the disease; these medications may cause retinopathy.

   5. Severe forms of the disease require **immunosuppressive therapy** with cyclophosphamide (which may cause bone marrow suppression, bladder carcinoma, or myelo- and lymphoproliferative malignancies) or azathioprine (which is less toxic). *[handwritten: Hemorrhagic cystitis   AZA]*

   [handwritten: 6. Cyclosporine A (CsA): renal disease is the indication]

V. SYSTEMIC SCLEROSIS (SCLERODERMA)

A. **General characteristics**

   1. **Systemic sclerosis** is a generalized disorder of connective tissue.

   2. **Inflammation and fibrosis** with small vessel obliteration affect skin, blood vessels, musculoskeletal system, GI tract, lungs, heart, and kidneys.

   3. Two clinical syndromes exist:

   a. **Diffuse systemic sclerosis** is characterized by widespread proximal skin involvement and early visceral involvement.

   b. **CREST syndrome** is characterized by subcutaneous calcinosis, Raynaud's phenomenon, esophageal dysmotility, sclerodactyly, and telangiectasia (visceral involvement is less common, and skin involvement is distal).

   4. **Age of onset** is between 30 and 60 years.

B. Clinical features

1. Disease usually begins with **Raynaud's phenomenon** (vasospasm in hands or feet due to cold that produces triphasic color change from pallor to cyanosis to hyperemia), **swelling of the hands,** or **distal polyarthralgias.**

2. **Thickening of the skin** occurs several months after initial signs and symptoms.
   a. Areas of **hypo- and hyperpigmentation,** loss of normal **skinfolds,** and **shiny skin** are common.
   b. **Telangiectasias** are present on the fingers, face, lips, and tongue.
   c. **Subcutaneous calcinosis** develops late in the CREST syndrome in the fingers, forearms, legs, and knees.

3. **Musculoskeletal** signs and symptoms include palpable friction over extensor surfaces, polyarthritis affecting both small and large joints, and muscle atrophy.

4. Common **GI** signs and symptoms include distal esophageal motor dysfunction, which leads to dysphagia for solid foods and reflux esophagitis; small bowel hypomotility is not uncommon, producing diarrhea, malabsorption and, occasionally, bacterial overgrowth syndrome.

5. **Pulmonary** signs and symptoms include shortness of breath on exertion secondary to pulmonary fibrosis, but pleuritis is uncommon (unlike SLE).

6. **Cardiac** signs and symptoms are less common, but arrhythmias and congestive heart failure (CHF) may occur; pericarditis is rare (unlike SLE).

7. **Renal** involvement is the leading cause of death in these patients; fibrosis of renal arterioles leads to malignant arterial hypertension and microangiopathic hemolytic anemia.

C. Laboratory findings

1. **Results** of routine laboratory tests are usually **normal.**

2. **Serum analysis** indicates positive test results for ANAs (not specific); anticentromere antibodies (if present, they are more diagnostic than are positive results for ANAs); hypocomplementemia and anti-dsDNA are rare (in contrast to SLE).

3. **Radiography**
   a. Barium esophagrams can effectively show **dysmotility and reflux.**
   b. **Osteopenia** is usually the only bony abnormality associated with systemic sclerosis.

D. Treatment

1. **Frequent evaluations** are necessary to assess the multiple systems affected by this disease, for example, barium swallows to assess esophageal motility; pulmonary function tests, cardiac ultrasound, and Holter monitoring to assess ventricular function and rhythm disturbances; and routine urinalysis to assess renal function.

2. **Penicillamine** inhibits collagen cross-linking, which leads to decreased skin thickening.

3. **Captopril** is effective in treating renal hypertensive disease.

4. **Calcium channel blockers** may provide relief of **Raynaud's phenomenon.**

5. **Corticosteroids** are generally not effective except for the treatment of polymyositis and pulmonary complications.

6. **Sucralfate** and **ranitidine** may be beneficial for the symptoms of esophageal

reflux, whereas **metoclopramide** (a smooth muscle stimulant) may improve intestinal motility.

VI. POLYMYOSITIS AND DERMATOMYOSITIS

A. General characteristics

1. Polymyositis and dermatomyositis are **inflammatory myopathies.**

2. A cardinal sign of dermatomyositis is a **characteristic rash.**

B. Clinical features

1. **Symmetric proximal muscle weakness** occurs after an insidious onset of malaise, weakness, and weight loss.

2. **Neck flexion weakness** is also present.

3. **Facial or ocular weakness** is not present (unlike myasthenia gravis).

4. Affected **muscles** may be **tender on palpation.**

5. Dermatomyositis is associated with **erythematous** smooth or scaly **patches** over elbows, knees, and medial malleoli, as well as **heliotrope eyelids** (violet discoloration of the eyelids).

6. Cardiac involvement may lead to **arrhythmias or CHF.**

7. **Swallowing difficulties** (dysphagia) are not uncommon.

C. Laboratory findings

1. Results of **routine laboratory tests** are usually **normal.**

2. **Serum analysis** indicates elevated levels of creatine kinase, lactate dehydrogenase (LDH), and aldolase; test results for ANAs are negative.

3. **Electromyography (EMG)** and **nerve conduction studies** help exclude denervating muscle diseases from the differential diagnosis.

D. Treatment

1. **High-dose oral corticosteroids** are prescribed for a 3-month trial period.

2. **Azathioprine, cyclophosphamide,** and **methotrexate** are second-line agents.

3. **Hydroxycloroquine** may be beneficial for resistant skin manifestations.

VII. SJÖGREN'S SYNDROME

A. General characteristics

1. Sjögren's syndrome is an inflammation and destruction of salivary and lacrimal glands.

2. The disease may be **primary** (an isolated condition) **or secondary** (usually associated with RA or SLE).

3. Sjögren's syndrome primarily affects **women in their 50s.**

B. Clinical features

1. The disease is characterized by the insidious onset of **dry eyes** (keratoconjunctivitis sicca), which creates a gritty sensation, or **dry mouth** (xerostomia), which

increases frequency of dental caries and creates difficulties in chewing and swallowing.

2. In time, **reduced visual acuity** and **photosensitivity** occur.

3. **Dryness** of the **nasopharynx** and **tracheobronchial tree** may lead to epistaxis, hoarseness, and bronchitis.

4. **Salivary gland enlargement** may occur.

5. **Constipation** and **pancreatic insufficiency** may occur due to mucosal gland involvement of these organs.

6. The disease is **strongly associated with lymphoma.**

C. **Laboratory findings**

1. **Hematologic studies** indicate normochromic-normocytic anemia and leukopenia; mild eosinophilia is seen in approximately one third of patients.

2. **Serum analysis** indicates the following:
a. Results of **tests for rheumatoid factor and ANAs** are often positive, but are not specific for Sjögren's disease.
b. **Anti-nucleoprotein** (anti-La) **antibodies** are fairly specific to the disease.
c. **Salivary gland biopsy** and a **consistent ophthalmologic examination** confirm the diagnosis.

D. **Treatment**

1. **Artificial tears for xerophthalmia** should be prescribed; topical corticosteroids should be avoided because they may cause corneal thinning.

2. **Xerostomia** can be **relieved with water,** and **scrupulous dental care** is necessary.

3. Treatment with **cyclophosphamide** and **corticosteroids** is reserved for patients who have severe disease.

VIII. VASCULITIC SYNDROMES

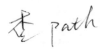

A. **General characteristics**

1. The **main pathologic feature** of these diseases is **inflammation of blood vessels.**

2. Common vasculitic syndromes discussed here include hypersensitivity angiitis, Henoch-Schönlein purpura, Churg-Strauss syndrome, polyarteritis nodosa, Wegener's granulomatosis, Goodpasture's syndrome, and giant cell arteritis.

B. **Hypersensitivity angiitis**

1. **General characteristics**
a. Hypersensitivity angiitis is the **most common form of vasculitis.**
b. The disease is localized to **skin involvement.**
c. **Infiltration of dermal capillaries** with PMNs occurs.
d. The disease tends to occur **following drug exposure.**

2. **Clinical features**
a. **Fever and arthralgias** may occur.
b. **Palpable purpura** is the primary skin feature, usually first seen on the lower extremities.

3. Laboratory findings
   a. **Skin biopsy** is the only diagnostic test.
   b. **Serum complement levels** may be **low or normal.**

4. Treatment
   a. The **causative agent** should be **discontinued.**
   b. **Corticosteroids** are useful in treating widespread disease.

C. Henoch-Schönlein purpura

1. General characteristics
   a. Henoch-Schönlein purpura is also known as **anaphylactoid or allergic purpura.**
   b. The disease occurs in **children** or **young adults.**
   c. The disease occurs **secondary to streptococcal infections, insect stings,** or administration of **drugs.**

2. Clinical features
   a. First signs of the disease are **palpable purpura** on the lower extremities, which may coalesce and ulcerate; purpura subsides in several weeks.
   b. **Abdominal pain,** upper or lower **GI bleeding,** and **lower extremity arthritis** may occur with the skin lesions or afterward; these signs and symptoms subside spontaneously.
   c. **Renal involvement** occurs in more than half of patients and is self-limiting.

3. Laboratory findings
   a. **Hematologic studies** indicate mild anemia, leukocytosis, and elevated ESR.
   b. **Urinalysis** indicates hematuria, red blood cell casts, and proteinuria, which indicate renal involvement.
   c. The presence of **IgA in tissue biopsy** confirms the diagnosis in patients who have appropriate symptomatology.

4. Treatment
   a. Therapy is **supportive for mild disease.**
   b. **Corticosteroids** are prescribed **for treating arthralgias** and **renal disease.**

D. Churg-Strauss syndrome

1. General characteristics
   a. Churg-Strauss syndrome is characterized by the **triad of asthma or allergic rhinitis, peripheral eosinophilia,** and **systemic vasculitis.**
   b. The disease **primarily affects men.**

2. Clinical features
   a. Allergic rhinitis usually precedes asthma.
   b. **Second phase** of the disease involves eosinophilic tissue infiltration.
   c. **Third phase** is characterized by systemic necrotizing vasculitis, weight loss, and fever.
   d. Vasculitis leads to nonprogressive glomerulonephritis, palpable purpura, and a nondeforming arthritis.

3. Laboratory findings
   a. **Hematologic studies** indicate leukocytosis with + + eosinophils, elevated levels of serum IgE, and normochromic anemia.
   b. **Tissue biopsy** reveals small-vessel vasculitis and eosinophilic infiltration.
   c. **Visceral angiography** may reveal tortuous vessels with areas of obliteration or partial occlusion.

4. Treatment
   a. **Systemic corticosteroids** are usually sufficient.
   b. **Azathioprine or cyclophosphamide** may be necessary to treat unremitting disease or to allow for tapering of corticosteroids.

E. **Polyarteritis nodosa**

1. **General characteristics**
   a. Polyarteritis nodosa involves medium-sized muscular arteries that form aneurysms and areas of occlusion.
   b. The disease **primarily affects middle-aged men.**
   c. The disease commonly affects skin, joints, nerves, GI tract, and kidneys.

2. **Clinical features**
   a. **Fever, malaise,** and **weight loss** occur frequently.
   b. **Seventy percent** of patients have **renal involvement,** which may lead to renal insufficiency and hypertension.
   c. **Peripheral neuropathy** occurs in 50% to 70% of patients, beginning with **sudden radicular pain** and **paresthesias,** followed by **motor deficits** involving that peripheral nerve.
   d. In the **skin,** palpable purpura, ulcerations, and digital tip infarcts may occur.
   e. In the joints, **nondeforming arthritis** involving any number of joints may occur.
   f. GI signs and symptoms include generalized **abdominal pain** and **distension,** which is suggestive of mesenteric artery involvement and may lead to obstruction, perforation, and GI bleeds.
   g. **Rupture of aneurysms** may lead to **hemorrhagic shock** and **death.**

3. **Laboratory findings**
   a. **Hematologic studies** indicate elevated ESR, leukocytosis, thrombocytosis, and anemia (from blood loss or renal failure).
   b. **Serum analysis** indicates hepatitis B surface antigen in 10% to 50% of patients and hypocomplementemia (C3 and C4) in one fourth of patients.
   c. **Urinalysis** reveals proteinuria, hematuria, and red blood cell casts, which indicate renal involvement.
   d. **Tissue biopsy** reveals vasculitis.
   e. **Visceral angiography** reveals microaneurysms and narrowing of segmental arteries.

4. **Treatment** consists of a combination of **steroid and immunosuppressive therapy** (cyclophosphamide).

F. **Wegener's granulomatosis**

1. **General characteristics**
   a. Wegener's granulomatosis **involves medium and small arteries.**
   b. The disease is characterized by **granulomatous vasculitis** of the upper and lower respiratory tract and a **necrotizing glomerulonephritis.**
   c. The disease **primarily affects middle-aged men.**

2. **Clinical features**
   a. Fever, anorexia, and weight loss are common.
   b. **Ulcerations of respiratory tract mucosa** lead to **chronic purulent sinusitis** and **saddle-nose deformity,** as well as pneumonitis, cavity formation, cough, and hemoptysis.
   c. Progressive renal disease **can be fatal.**
   d. **Eye inflammation with episcleritis** occurs in over half of patients.

    e. GI tract and peripheral nerves are less commonly involved (unlike polyarteritis nodosa).

  3. **Laboratory findings**

    a. **Hematologic studies** indicate normochromic anemia, leukocytosis without eosinophilia, and thrombocytosis.

    b. **Serum analysis** indicates elevated IgE and IgA levels; positive results for PMN cytoplasm (this result is fairly specific for active disease).

    c. **Urinalysis** reveals red blood cell casts, proteinuria, and hematuria, which indicate glomerular disease.

  4. **Treatment** consists of combined **corticosteroid and cyclophosphamide therapy,** which has markedly improved the outcome of this disease.

G. **Goodpasture's syndrome** : *young man*

  1. **General characteristics**

    a. Goodpasture's syndrome is characterized by **pulmonary hemorrhage** and **glomerulonephritis.**

    b. **Antiglomerular basement membrane antibodies** are present and may also **bind to lung basement membranes,** which gives rise to disease manifestations.

    c. The disease **primarily affects young men.**

  2. **Clinical features** include an initial **flulike prodrome,** followed by renal and lung manifestations (**cough** and **hemoptysis**).

  3. **Laboratory findings**

    a. **Hematologic studies** indicate microcytic, hypochromic anemia and low serum iron levels.

    b. **Urinalysis** reveals proteinuria, hematuria, and red blood cell casts, which indicate glomerular involvement.

    c. **Immunohistologic studies** of renal biopsy tissue show linear deposits of antibodies along the glomerular basement membrane.

    d. **Lung biopsy** reveals alveolar hemorrhage and hemosiderosis; **immunologic studies** show linear deposits of antibodies along alveolar basement membrane.

  4. **Treatment**

    a. **High-dose corticosteroids, cytotoxic drugs,** and occasionally, **plasmapheresis** are prescribed.

    b. **Hemodialysis** may be necessary.

H. **Giant cell arteritis** *polymyalgia rheumatica.*

  1. **General characteristics**

    a. Giant cell arteritis is a granulomatous vasculitis that **affects persons older than 50 years** of age.

    b. The disease may coexist with **polymyalgia rheumatica** (characterized by aching extremities, stiffness, fatigue, and headache).

  2. **Clinical features** *jaw, tongue,*

    a. **Symptoms** include those of **claudication** (pain, pallor, paresthesias, pulselessness); **headache; visual changes;** and **scalp tenderness.**

    b. **Common sites of claudication** include jaw (indicating temporal arteritis), tongue, and extremities.

    c. **Visual changes** include blurring, ptosis, diplopia, and partial or complete blindness (due to ophthalmic vessel arteritis).

    d. New onset of headache in an elderly person suggests the diagnosis.

    e. Tenderness over the **affected portion of the temporal artery** may be elicited, and this area should undergo **biopsy immediately** because of the **risk of blindness.**

3. Laboratory findings

    a. **Hematologic studies** indicate normochromic anemia, leukocytosis, thrombocytosis, and elevated ESR (which is highly suggestive of the diagnosis in an elderly person who has the appropriate symptoms).

    b. **Temporal arteriography** often gives **false-positive results;** therefore, **biopsy** remains the **mainstay of diagnosis.**

4. **Treatment** consists of **corticosteroids,** which should be administered if the diagnosis is highly suspected on the basis of clinical symptoms, to **avert** the complication of **blindness** (even if biopsy has not yet been performed).

2

Endocrinologic and Metabolic Disorders

I. DISORDERS OF THE PITUITARY GLAND

A. General characteristics

   1. **Diseases** may affect the anterior and/or posterior pituitary gland.

   2. **Anterior pituitary diseases** include pituitary tumors, anterior pituitary hypofunction, and pituitary hyperfunction.

   3. **Posterior pituitary diseases** include diabetes insipidus and syndrome of inappropriate antidiuretic hormone secretion (SIADH).

B. Pituitary tumors

   1. General characteristics
      a. Pituitary tumors account for **10% of intracranial tumors.**
      b. Pituitary tumors **may be nonfunctioning.**
      c. **Functioning tumors** are usually chromophobic adenomas that produce adrenocorticotropic hormone (**ACTH**), growth hormone (**GH**), or prolactin (**PRL**).
      d. **Secretion of** thyroid-stimulating hormone (**TSH**), follicle-stimulating hormone (**FSH**), or luteinizing hormone (**LH**) is **rare.**

   2. Clinical features
      a. Patients who have pituitary tumors may be seen with **headache** or **visual disturbance** (bitemporal hemianopia).
      b. Patients who have functioning tumors may be seen with **endocrinologic manifestations,** for example, galactorrhea-amenorrhea (PRL-secreting tumor), acromegaly (GH-secreting tumor), Cushing's syndrome (ACTH-secreting tumor).
      c. Patients who have nonfunctioning tumors may be seen with **signs and symptoms of anterior pituitary hypofunction** (see I C).

   3. Laboratory findings
      a. Computed tomography (**CT**) scans with contrast medium are useful in **diagnosing** adenomas < 10 mm in diameter (**microadenomas**).
      b. **Growth hormone, prolactin, or ACTH** levels are often **elevated** even when diagnostic imaging cannot visualize the tumor.

   4. Treatment
      a. **Surgical removal** of the tumor is indicated if neurologic symptoms or syndromes of excess hormone production are present.

  b. Radiotherapy alone or as an adjunct to surgery often reduces tumor size, but often results in hypopituitarism.

  c. Bromocriptine (dopamine agonist) often sufficiently controls small PRL-secreting adenomas.

  d. In nonfunctioning tumors, **hormonal replacement** is required.

C. Anterior pituitary hypofunction

  1. General characteristics

  a. Anterior pituitary hypofunction may occur secondary to destruction of the pituitary by a nonfunctioning pituitary tumor.

  b. The disease may also occur secondary to infarction resulting from hypotension during childbirth (Sheehan's syndrome), or surgical removal of the pituitary gland.

  2. Clinical features

  a. GH deficiency causes growth failure if disease occurs during childhood, but adults are not affected by GH deficiency.

  b. LH/FSH deficiency causes amenorrhea and breast atrophy in women, genital atrophy, and loss of potency and libido in men.

  c. TSH deficiency causes signs and symptoms associated with hypothyroidism (see II C).

  d. ACTH deficiency causes secondary adrenal insufficiency (which differs clinically from primary adrenal insufficiency).

   (1) Hyperpigmentation **does not** occur as in primary adrenal insufficiency because ACTH levels are decreased.

   (2) Decreased serum sodium and increased serum potassium levels are not severe in secondary adrenal insufficiency because aldosterone secretion is largely dependent upon the renin-angiotensin system rather than ACTH.

   (3) Hyponatremia may occur secondary to decreased cortisol levels, which is necessary for free water excretion.

  e. PRL deficiency causes no clinical manifestations except in Sheehan's syndrome, in which it results in postpartum failure of lactation.

  3. Laboratory findings

  a. The **diagnosis** is established by low levels of target organ hormones (cortisol, thyroxine, testosterone, estrogen) and an absence of compensatory increases in corresponding pituitary hormones (ACTH, TSH, FSH/LH).

  b. The **metyrapone test,** which blocks cortisol production, is used to evaluate pituitary ACTH production.

  c. Necessary **GH secretion** may be assessed by the insulin-induced hypoglycemia test; this test stimulates pituitary GH release in response to hypoglycemia induced by an injection of regular insulin.

  4. Treatment

  a. An **underlying cause** for hypopituitarism (e.g., a tumor) must be ruled out.

  b. GH replacement is necessary only in affected children.

  c. PRL replacement is generally unnecessary.

  d. Thyroxine and cortisol are necessary: cortisol should be given before or with thyroxine in order to prevent an addisonian crisis (thyroxine alone causes increased clearance of endogenous glucocorticoids).

  e. Testosterone is indicated to restore libido and potency in men, and **estrogen-progesterone** is indicated to restore menstrual function in women.

D. Pituitary hyperfunction

  1. General characteristics

  a. Pituitary hyperfunction primarily presents as **hyperprolactinemia** or **acromegaly/gigantism.**

  b. Because PRL secretion is inhibited by hypothalamic dopamine, damage to the pituitary stalk or inhibition of dopamine will produce hyperprolactinemia (e.g., phenothiazines, which act as dopamine antagonists, will cause hyperprolactinemia).

 2. Clinical features

  a. In women, hyperprolactinemia produces persistent **galactorrhea** (unprovoked by breast stimulation) and **amenorrhea;** in men, it may also produce galactorrhea, but **loss of libido** and **impotence** are more common.

  b. Before adulthood, **gigantism** occurs because of increased linear growth of bones before epiphyseal closure.

  c. **Acromegaly** occurs after epiphyseal closure and is associated with thickening of skin, acral enlargement (enlargement of fingers and toes), coarsening and enlargement of facial features, and frontal bossing.

  d. **Impaired glucose tolerance** occurs as a result of the glucose-elevating effect of GH; overt diabetes is uncommon.

  e. **GH** increases renal phosphate reabsorption, which results in hyperphosphatemia.

 3. Laboratory findings

  a. Hyperprolactinemia is confirmed by PRL levels > 150 ng/dl (normal < 20 ng/dl); these levels suggest PRL-secreting adenoma.

   (1) PRL levels < 150 ng/dl suggest non-neoplastic causes (e.g., drugs, stress, pituitary stalk lesion, hypothyroidism).

   (2) Multiple tests of PRL levels may be necessary because PRL may be secreted intermittently.

  b. Gigantism/acromegaly can be confirmed by GH levels > 10 ng/ml under basal conditions (before rising from bed in the morning); the diagnosis is more conclusive if GH is not suppressed to < 5 ng/ml within 2 hours of ingestion of 100 g of glucose.

 4. Treatment

  a. Treatment of hyperprolactinemia includes:

   (1) Initial trial of **bromocriptine** for patients who have smaller PRL-secreting tumors

   (2) **Transsphenoidal microsurgery** for larger tumors that produce neurologic symptoms (surgery causes hypopituitarism less frequently than radiotherapy)

  b. Treatment for gigantism/acromegaly includes **pituitary adenomectomy** for small tumors; adenomectomy is less effective in reducing GH levels to normal when tumors are large.

   (1) **Radiotherapy** reduces GH levels over a period of years and therefore is not as effective as adenomectomy.

   (2) **Bromocriptine** may be used as an adjunct to radiotherapy.

E. Diabetes insipidus (DI)

 1. General characteristics

  a. Diabetes insipidus is caused by an impaired urinary concentrating mechanism.

  b. The disease may occur because renal distal tubules fail to respond to ADH (antidiuretic hormone)(nephrogenic DI) or because ADH (central DI) is lacking.

  c. **Fifty percent** of cases are **idiopathic.**

  d. Head trauma, neurosurgical procedures, and brain tumors account for the remainder of cases.

Table 2-1
Results of Water Deprivation Test for Diabetes Insipidus (DI)

Patient Type	Increase in [Urine] with Dehydration	Further Response to ADH
Normal	Yes	None
Nephrogenic DI	None	None
Central DI	None	Yes

ADH = antidiuretic hormone.

   2. Clinical features
     a. **Polyuria** is a prominent symptom (3–15 L/d is not uncommon).
     b. Patients report **excessive thirst,** which is a physiologic response to water loss.

   3. Laboratory findings
     a. Urine is dilute with specific gravity < 1.010 and osmolality < 300 mOsm/kg.
     b. **Serum osmolality** is high or normal (> 280 mOsm/kg) in DI secondary to excess water loss; in psychogenic polydypsia, serum osmolality tends to be < 280 mOsm/kg because of excess water intake.
     c. **Water deprivation test**
       (1) Normally, overnight water restriction stimulates ADH release, which leads to a more concentrated urine.
       (2) Once urine osmolality stabilizes, ADH is injected into the patient, and the urine osmolality is reassessed; Table 2-1 lists results of the water deprivation tests.

   4. Treatment
     a. In acute central DI (e.g., head injuries), **aqueous vasopressin** acts rapidly.
     b. For partial ADH deficiency, **chlorpropamide** (an oral hypoglycemic agent) will potentiate the effects of ADH on the renal tubule.
     c. **Thiazide diuretics** are the only treatment for nephrogenic DI.

F. **SIADH**

   1. General characteristics
     a. **Excess ADH** may be produced by malignant tumors (e.g., oat cell carcinoma of the lung); pulmonary diseases (e.g., pneumonia, tuberculosis); central nervous system (CNS) disorders (e.g., stroke, head injury); or drugs (e.g., chlorpropamide, carbamazepine).
     b. SIADH causes increased free water retention.
       (1) The body compensates for the increased water retention through **natriuresis.**
       (2) This compensation results in only mild volume expansion and hyponatremia.

   2. **Clinical features** of SIADH are those of hyponatremia, such as lethargy, confusion, headache, focal neurologic abnormalities, convulsions, and coma.

   3. Laboratory findings
     a. **Hyponatremia** is indicated by a serum Na^+ level < 135 mmol/L; hyponatremia is critical if serum Na^+ level falls acutely below 125 mmol/L.
     b. **Urinary sodium excretion** continues despite hyponatremia (> 20 mmol/day) and U_{osm} (urine osmolality) > S_{osm} (serum osmolality).

4. Treatment
   a. It is necessary to treat the underlying cause of SIADH.
   b. **Fluid restriction** of 500 to 1000 ml/day will effectively correct hyponatremia.
   c. If serum sodium < 120 mmol/L, **hypertonic saline** (3%–5%) should be used as a temporizing measure.
   d. **Demeclocycline** inhibits the effects of ADH on renal tubules (which is a side effect), thereby minimizing free water reabsorption.

II. DISORDERS OF THE THYROID GLAND

A. Diseases of the thyroid gland include hyperthyroidism, hypothyroidism, thyroiditis, thyroid cancer, and thyroid nodules.

B. Hyperthyroidism

1. General characteristics
   a. **Graves' disease** (diffuse toxic goiter) is the most common form of hyperthyroidism.
   (1) Graves' disease is an autoimmune disorder in which antibodies to TSH are produced.
   (2) Production of TSH antibodies leads to diffuse enlargement and thyroid hormone (TH) production.
   b. **Plummer's disease** (nodular toxic goiter) affects older individuals.
   (1) This disease is characterized by discrete areas of autonomously **hyperfunctioning thyroid gland.**
   (2) **Normal thyroid tissue functions** are **suppressed** because of negative feedback on TSH.
   c. **Subacute thyroiditis** is another type of hyperthyroidism; (see thyroiditis, II D).
   d. **Factitious hyperthyroidism** is caused by excessive ingestion of TH by patients.

2. Clinical features
   a. **Metabolic changes** include elevated metabolic rate, weight loss, increased appetite, sweating, and heat intolerance.
   b. **Cardiovascular signs and symptoms** include widened pulse pressure, sinus tachycardia, atrial fibrillation (producing palpitations), and premature ventricular complexes.
   c. **Gastrointestinal (GI) signs and symptoms** include loose stools and diarrhea.
   d. **Skin** is warm and moist because of peripheral vasodilation and perspiration; **hair** becomes thin and fine.
   e. **CNS signs and symptoms** include fine tremor, emotional lability and restlessness, and brisk return phase of deep tendon reflexes.
   f. **Musculoskeletal signs and symptoms** include muscle weakness and fatigue.
   g. **Ophthalmopathy** includes exophthalmos (in Graves' disease only), lid lag (on downward gaze), lid retraction, tearing, irritation, pain, and diplopia.
   h. A **thyroid storm** is a sudden exacerbation of hyperthyroidism characterized by marked fever, agitation, and tachycardia progressing to coma and hypotension.
   i. In Graves' disease, a uniformly enlarged thyroid gland is palpable, whereas in Plummer's disease, one or more nodules may be palpable.

3. Laboratory findings
   a. Elevated serum levels of T_3 and T_4 (thyroid hormones) **with low TSH** indicate hyperthyroidism.
   b. **Radioactive iodine uptake test** measures uptake of iodine by the thyroid gland,

which indicates functional state; in factitious hyperthyroidism, thyroid uptake is decreased because exogenous TH suppresses the gland's function.

    c. In the **T_3 resin uptake test,** the patient's serum is combined with radiolabeled T_3 and a T_3-binder.

        (1) If excess T_3 is present, an increased amount of T_3 will bind to the binder (normal T_3 resin uptake is approximately 30%).

        (2) Elevated T_3 resin uptake indicates hyperthyroidism.

4. Treatment

    a. Thirty percent of patients who have Graves' disease will go into spontaneous remission within 2 years; therefore, **cautious medical management** is preferred to total thyroid ablation (which causes hypothyroidism).

    b. **Beta-blockers** can be used initially to stabilize the patient's cardiovascular function.

    c. **Methimazole** and **propylthiouracil** (PTU) inhibit TH production, but effects are not seen for weeks to months because large endogenous storage pools of hormone are present.

        (1) PTU also inhibits peripheral conversion of T_4 to T_3; the drug dose is tapered and discontinued after 1 to 2 years.

        (2) PTU is often used in younger patients with mild disease who have a better chance of remission.

        (3) Side effects of PTU include skin rash in 3% to 5% of patients and agranulocytosis in <0.5% of patients.

    d. **Subtotal thyroidectomy** offers rapid therapy with a high cure rate and eliminates the need for long-term patient compliance with medications.

        (1) **Complications** include recurrent laryngeal nerve paralysis, hypothyroidism, hypoparathyroidism, or precipitation of thyroid storm preoperatively.

        (2) Subtotal thyroidectomy is reserved for patients who have large goiters and severe disease or for those who are unlikely to be compliant with medication.

    e. **Radioactive iodine therapy** involves a single dose of iodine 131.

        (1) **Single-dose radiotherapy** produces euthyroidism in 75% of Graves' disease patients (during a 6-week period).

        (2) Radiotherapy often results in **subsequent hypothyroidism;** therefore, it is generally used in patients older than 40 years of age.

C. Hypothyroidism

1. General characteristics

    a. Hypothyroidism is most commonly caused by **Hashimoto's** (chronic) **thyroiditis** (see II D 3).

    b. **Idiopathic atrophy** (often associated with antithyroid antibodies) is also common.

    c. Hypothyroidism frequently develops as a result of treatment for Graves' hyperthyroidism.

    d. **Drugs** such as lithium, iodide, and amiodarone have been reported to cause hyperthyroidism as well.

    e. Hypothyroidism may be secondary to hypothalamic-pituitary dysfunction.

    f. **Iodine deficiency** is an uncommon cause in developed countries, but may be more common in other areas of the world.

2. Clinical features

    a. **Symptoms** include weakness, lethargy, slowness of thought and speech, sleepiness, and fatigue.

   b. **Signs** include puffy appearance, nonpitting edema (myxedema), dry skin, coarse hair, and cold intolerance.

   c. Patients report **diminished appetite** but experience **mild weight gain** (due to decreased metabolic rate) and **constipation.**

   d. **Edema of the larynx and middle ear** leads to voice changes and hearing loss.

   e. **Menstrual irregularities** may also occur and are associated with anovulatory cycles.

   f. **Slow return phase of deep tendon reflexes** is observed.

   g. Myxedema coma

   (1) Is caused by severe hypothyroidism, which is triggered by stress, such as infection, alcohol, or drugs

   (2) Leads to respiratory insufficiency, hypothermia, hypoglycemia, sluggish cerebral perfusion, and coma

   (3) Has a significant mortality rate

3. **Laboratory findings**

   a. **Serum levels of T_3, T_4, and T_3-resin uptake** are decreased.

   b. **Radioactive iodine uptake** is decreased.

   c. In primary hypothyroidism, **serum TSH** is increased.

4. **Treatment**

   a. **L-thyroxine** is the agent of choice (maintenance dose is 0.1 to 0.15 mg/day in the adult; half dose in the elderly).

   b. Treatment must be started slowly because patients who have severe disease have increased sensitivity to TH.

   c. Myxedema coma must be treated rapidly despite the risks associated with sudden hormone replacement (0.5 mg intravenous bolus).

   d. Therapy adequacy is determined by a return of TSH and serum thyroid hormones to normal levels.

D. **Thyroiditis**

1. Thyroiditis is a **group of disorders** consisting predominantly of subacute thyroiditis (de Quervain's thyroiditis), Hashimoto's (chronic) thyroiditis, and painless thyroiditis.

2. **Subacute thyroiditis**

   a. Subacute thyroiditis has a **viral etiology** (mumps or coxsackievirus).

   b. **Clinical features**

   (1) Patients report a 1- to 2-week prodrome of malaise, upper respiratory tract symptoms, and fever.

   (2) The thyroid gland becomes enlarged (goiter), firm, and painful.

   (3) Symptoms of hyperthyroidism occur as a result of leakage of TH from the inflamed gland.

   (4) Disease lasts for weeks to months and then subsides; gland returns to normal size.

   c. **Laboratory findings**

   (1) T_3 and T_4 levels are elevated, and radioactive iodine uptake is decreased; these results are due to leakage of TH from the gland rather than hyperfunction of the gland.

   (2) TSH levels are low because of excess thyroid hormone.

   d. **Treatment**

   (1) Symptomatic treatment is sufficient until disease remits.

   (2) Nonsteroidal anti-inflammatory drugs (**NSAIDs**) relieve pain of inflammation, whereas β-blocking agents are used to relieve symptoms of hyperthyroidism.

(3) PTU and **methimazole** are not useful because excess hormone is not produced.

3. Hashimoto's thyroiditis
  a. General characteristics
    (1) Hashimoto's thyroiditis is an **autoimmune disease** in which antithyroid antibodies are produced.
    (2) The disease **primarily affects women.**
  b. Clinical features
    (1) Autoimmune damage leads to **thyroid fibrosis and enlargement** (goiter).
    (2) Pain and tenderness of the gland sometimes occur.
    (3) Patients often report **symptoms of hypothyroidism.**
  c. Laboratory findings
    (1) Antithyroid antibodies are present in serum.
    (2) Serum T₃ and T₄ levels are decreased, and **serum TSH level** is increased if hypothyroidism occurs.
  d. Treatment
    (1) L-thyroxine is necessary in the hypothyroid patient.
    (2) L-thyroxine also decreases the size of the goiter, which makes this thyroid hormone useful therapy in the euthyroid patient who has thyroid enlargement.

4. Painless thyroiditis (lymphocytic thyroiditis)
  a. Clinical features
    (1) Painless thyroiditis is similar to subacute thyroiditis; that is, it is a **self-limiting hyperthyroidism** secondary to inflammatory damage (lymphocytic infiltration), which produces thyroid enlargement.
    (2) Hyperthyroidism, goiter, and **absence of pain** also suggest the diagnosis of Graves' disease, which may lead to inappropriate therapy.
  b. Laboratory findings
    (1) Radioactive iodine uptake is **decreased** in painless thyroiditis because the thyroid gland is damaged (as in subacute thyroiditis), but uptake is **increased** in Graves' disease.
    (2) T_3 and T_4 levels are elevated, and TSH level is increased in serum.
  c. Treatment
    (1) Symptomatic therapy is given with **β-blockers** until remission occurs.
    (2) Antithyroid drugs are not useful.

E. Thyroid cancer

  1. General characteristics
    a. Thyroid cancer is **associated with previous radiotherapy to the neck.**
    b. A **genetic association** has been found **to medullary carcinoma** of the thyroid.
    c. Thyroid cancer often presents as a **solitary thyroid nodule** rather than multiple nodules.

  2. Types of thyroid cancer include:
    a. Papillary carcinoma
      (1) Papillary carcinoma accounts for **60% of all thyroid cancers.**
      (2) This cancer usually **affects persons younger than 40** years of age.
      (3) The cancer is **slow growing** and remains **localized** for years; the cancer **then spreads** to regional lymph nodes.
      (4) Patients have **few recurrences after treatment.**
    b. Follicular carcinoma
      (1) Follicular carcinoma is the **second most common** type of **thyroid cancer.**

(2) Follicular carcinoma is **TSH-dependent** and looks and **functions like normal thyroid tissue.**
(3) This cancer **metastasizes to bone, brain, and lung.**
(4) **Ten-year survival rate** is 50%.
  c. Anaplastic carcinoma
(1) Anaplastic carcinoma accounts for **10% of thyroid cancers.**
(2) This type of thyroid cancer **primarily affects older patients.**
(3) The tumor is **aggressive,** with **early metastasis and death** within months.
  d. Medullary carcinoma
(1) Medullary carcinoma arises from parafollicular cells.
(2) The tumor can produce **calcitonin.**
(3) This cancer is **associated with** multiple endocrine neoplasia syndrome **(MEN type II).**

3. Treatment
  a. Papillary, follicular, and medullary carcinoma are first **surgically removed.**
  b. Because these tumors are TSH-sensitive, **L-thyroxine** is then administered indefinitely to suppress TSH.
  c. **Radioactive iodine therapy** is used to ablate distant metastases and any remaining thyroid gland tumor after surgery.

F. Thyroid nodules
  1. General characteristics
  a. Thyroid nodules are present in **up to 5% of the population.**
  b. **Ten to twenty percent** of nodules are **malignant;** the remainder may be cystic, colloid, hemorrhagic, or inflammatory.
  c. **Nodules** are **more likely malignant** when:
(1) They occur in **young men.**
(2) Patients report a **history of radiotherapy to the head or neck during childhood.**
(3) The **nodule grows rapidly,** and growth is **not suppressed by L-thyroxine therapy.**
(4) The nodule appears "cold" on a radioactive iodine scintiscan (i.e., no uptake). **Note: warm or hot nodules** are **rarely malignant.**
(5) The nodule appears **solid on ultrasound.**
  2. Diagnosis
  a. **Radioactive iodine scintigraphy** determines if the lesion is more likely to be malignant (i.e., cold), but this procedure is not diagnostic.
  b. **Fine-needle aspiration** is most diagnostic and is easily performed with little risk to the patient.
  3. Treatment
  a. **Surgery** is indicated if history and physical examination suggest malignancy, cytology is equivocal or malignant, or the nodule continues to grow despite thyroid hormone therapy.
  b. **Conservative management** and observation are indicated if the nodule is "warm," history and physical examination are not suspicious, and cytology is benign.

III. DISORDERS OF THE PARATHYROID GLAND

A. Primary hyperparathyroidism and hypercalcemia
  1. General characteristics
  a. Oversecretion of parathyroid hormone (PTH) causes **hypercalcemia.**
  b. Primary hyperparathyroidism **affects 1 in 1000 persons (primarily middle-aged and elderly women).**

c. Most cases are due to **parathyroid adenoma.**

d. Primary hyperparathyroidism may be associated with **MEN syndromes.**

e. **Secondary hyperparathyroidism** results from ongoing stimulation of the parathyroid glands due to low serum calcium, which is most commonly caused by **chronic renal failure** (decreased vitamin D hydroxylation).

2. Clinical features of hypercalcemia

a. In the renal system, increased serum calcium leads to **urinary calculi** and **nephrocalcinosis,** which may progress to **renal failure.**

b. **CNS signs and symptoms** include lethargy, stupor, fatigue, proximal myopathy and hypotonia, and coma.

c. **GI signs and symptoms** include anorexia, nausea, vomiting, constipation, and abdominal pain.

d. **Hypercalcemia** causes **osteitis fibrosa cystica,** which is characterized by bone pain, fractures, deformities, bone cysts, generalized osteopenia, and subperiosteal bone resorption in the phalanges.

3. Laboratory findings

a. **Serum analysis** indicates increased Ca^{2+} with elevated PTH levels, decreased PO_4^{2-} level, elevated alkaline phosphatase level (in patients who have significant bone disease), decreased HCO_3 level, and elevated Cl^- level (an effect of excess PTH).

b. **Urinalysis** may indicate hypercalciuria.

c. **Ultrasound and CT** may reveal parathyroid adenomas in more than half of cases; subperiosteal bone resorption of the phalanges is highly suggestive of the diagnosis.

4. Differential diagnosis of hypercalcemia

a. Differential diagnosis of hypercalcemia is **based on PTH levels.**

b. Disorders in which PTH levels are decreased are secondary causes of hypercalcemia and include:

(1) **Tumors with bone metastases** (e.g., breast, myeloma, lymphoma)

(2) **Tumors without bone metastases** in which a PTH-like substance is produced by the malignancy, such as squamous cell carcinoma of the lung or cervix and pancreatic carcinoma

(3) **Sarcoidosis,** which results in vitamin D_3 production within the granulomas and leads to hypercalcemia

(4) **Vitamin D intoxication**

(5) **Familial hypocalciuric hypercalcemia**

(6) **Hyperthyroidism,** which leads to increased bone turnover

(7) **Rhabdomyolysis**

(a) Initially, calcium and phosphate are deposited in damaged muscle.

(b) Calcium and phosphate then enter the blood as acute renal failure subsides, producing hypercalcemia (over 2 to 3 weeks).

5. Treatment

a. **Emergency therapy** is required if serum calcium levels rise above 13 to 15 mg/dl.

(1) **Diuresis with furosemide and intravenous saline** (5–10 L/day) increases renal calcium excretion.

(2) **Mithramycin** inhibits osteoclastic bone resorption, which reduces serum calcium.

(3) **Glucocorticoids** lower calcium absorption from the gut, which is effective in **sarcoidosis** and **vitamin D intoxication** only.

(4) Phosphate decreases serum calcium levels, but **calcium phosphate deposition in tissues** may occur.

   b. Surgical removal of parathyroid adenoma is indicated in patients who have elevated serum calcium levels (> 11.0 mg/dl).

   c. Medical therapy is indicated for patients who have mildly elevated serum calcium levels.

      (1) Increased fluid intake increases renal calcium excretion.

      (2) Oral phosphate can decrease serum calcium levels and usually does not produce calcium phosphate deposition in small doses.

      (3) Estrogen decreases bone resorption and may be beneficial in postmenopausal patients who have mild hypercalcemia.

B. Hypoparathyroidism and hypocalcemia

   1. General characteristics

      a. Hypoparathyroidism is most commonly **caused by surgical removal of the parathyroid glands** during a neck procedure.

      b. Idiopathic cases occur less commonly.

   2. Clinical features

      a. Latent tetany, which occurs with mild hypocalcemia, may manifest as muscular fatigue and weakness with circumoral paresthesias.

         (1) Patients exhibit **positive Chvostek's sign** (tapping anterior to the ear on the facial nerve elicits facial muscle contraction).

         (2) Patients exhibit **positive Trousseau's sign** (carpal tunnel spasm is induced by inflated blood pressure cuff on arm).

      b. Overt tetany, which occurs with severe hypocalcemia, manifests as muscle twitching and spasm progressing to laryngeal stridor and seizures.

      c. Long-term effects of hypocalcemia include brittle, ridged nails; dry skin; and enamel defects of teeth.

         (1) Calcification of basal ganglia may lead to parkinsonian signs and symptoms.

         (2) Calcification of lens leads to cataract formation.

   3. Differential diagnosis of hypocalcemia

      a. Hypoalbuminemia leads to decreased protein-bound serum calcium.

         (1) Decreased protein-bound serum calcium results in a decreased total serum calcium.

         (2) However, the **ionized fraction of serum calcium** is unchanged; therefore, no clinical manifestations of hypocalcemia occur (for every 1 g/L drop in serum albumin, serum calcium decreases by 0.8 mg/dl).

      b. In renal failure, **decreased 1,25-dihydroxyvitamin D_3** leads to decreased calcium absorption.

      c. Osteoblastic metastasis of lung, prostate, or breast cancers may cause rapid uptake of calcium by bone.

      d. Hypomagnesemia leads to decreased production of PTH and inhibits action of PTH and vitamin D on bone.

      e. In acute pancreatitis, an association with **hypocalcemia** has been established, but the cause remains uncertain.

         (1) Diabetic nephropathy commonly develops in insulin-dependent diabetes mellitus but rarely occurs in non-insulin-dependent diabetes mellitus.

         (2) Cerebral, coronary, and peripheral vascular disease occurs earlier and is more extensive than in the general population.

         (3) Symmetric distal polyneuropathy and paresthesias occur with loss of sensation in a **stocking-glove distribution,** which can lead to **neuro-pathic foot ulcers** or **Charcot's joints.**

    (4) **Autonomic neuropathies** may present as neurogenic bladder; urinary retention and urinary tract infections; gastroparesis; intermittent diarrhea and constipation; and orthostatic hypotension.

  4. **Laboratory findings**

    a. **Serum analysis** indicates low calcium and high phosphate levels, with a concomitantly decreased PTH level.

    b. **Radiography** indicates no specific changes.

  5. **Treatment**

    a. **PTH is not available** for treatment.

    b. Therapy consists of **replacement of serum calcium** orally or intravenously (if severe) along with vitamin D.

IV. Glucose homeostasis

  A. Diabetes mellitus

    1. **General characteristics**

      a. **Type I** (insulin-dependent diabetes mellitus [IDDM]) **affects young, lean individuals.**

        (1) Patients are insulin-dependent.

        (2) Patients are prone to diabetic ketoacidosis (DKA).

        (3) IDDM is human leukocyte antigen and autoimmune associated.

      b. **Type II** (non–insulin-dependent diabetes mellitus [NIDDM]) **affects obese, older individuals.**

        (1) Patients produce some insulin and are insulin-resistant.

        (2) Patients do not develop DKA.

        (3) NIDDM has a genetic association.

    2. **Clinical features**

      a. **Symptoms** include polyuria, polydipsia, blurred vision, and weight loss and weakness despite increased food intake.

      b. Patients have an increased frequency of **skin and urinary tract infections.**

      c. A **complication** of diabetes is retinopathy, which is most commonly associated with soft exudates, microaneurysms, and retinal hemorrhages.

    3. **Laboratory findings**

      a. **Persistent fasting blood sugar** < 140 mg/dl is diagnostic.

      b. **Glucose tolerance test** suggests diabetic tendencies if blood sugar (BS) > 140 mg/dl 2 hours after glucose challenge, and the test is diagnostic if BS > 200 mg/dl.

      c. **Glycosylated hemoglobin levels** reflect the degree of hyperglycemia during a period of 6 to 12 weeks and are thus a useful tool in monitoring therapy and compliance.

      d. **Urine glucose levels** are often variable and therefore not useful in diagnosis.

    4. **Treatment**

      a. Therapy for IDDM consists of **dietary management and insulin.**

        (1) The **recommended diet** should consist of 25% to 30% lipid, 50% to 60% carbohydrate, and 10% to 20% protein.

Table 2-2

Classification of Insulin Types

Insulin Type	Classification	Onset of Action (h)
Regular	Short-acting	<1 h
Isophane insulin	Intermediate-acting	2–3 h
Zinc (Lente) insulin	Intermediate-acting	2–3 h
Ultralente insulin	Long-acting	4–6 h

(2) Initially, patients take **one dose of intermediate insulin** (Table 2-2) before breakfast; serial serum glucose levels are measured before each meal and at bedtime.

(3) **If all serum glucose measurements are uniformly elevated** after beginning treatment, the morning dose of insulin is increased.

(4) **If only morning serum glucose levels are high,** a short-acting insulin dose may be added to the morning regimen.

(5) **If only evening serum glucose levels are high,** an intermediate-acting insulin dose may be added in the afternoon.

  b. **Therapy for NIDDM** consists of dietary management and may include oral hypoglycemic agents or insulin.

(1) **Dietary management** is of greatest importance and should emphasize weight loss.

(2) If dietary management results in insufficient control, **oral hypoglycemic agents** (e.g., chlorpropamide [may cause SIADH-like symptoms] or glyburide) **or insulin** is indicated.

B. Diabetic ketoacidosis (DKA)

1. General characteristics

  a. Diabetic ketoacidosis occurs in IDDM patients because of **stress** (e.g., infection, injury, alcohol) or **worsening glucose control,** which produces hyperglycemia → osmotic diuresis → dehydration and hyponatremia.

  b. **Insufficient insulin** → increased lipolysis → increased ketones → anion gap metabolic acidosis (see IV B 3 a) → compensatory respiratory alkalosis (hyperventilation).

2. Clinical features

  a. Patients exhibit a **decreased level of consciousness.**

  b. **Deep rapid breathing** (Kussmaul's respirations) occurs.

  c. **Acetone breath** is detected.

  d. **Signs of dehydration** are apparent, for example, dry mucous membranes and axillae, tachycardia, and postural hypotension.

3. Laboratory findings

  a. **Serum analysis** indicates hyperglycemia (glucose often > 500 mg/dl); elevated ketone levels (acetoacetate, acetone, β-hydroxybutyrate); and decreased serum bicarbonate level (HCO_3) [anion gap metabolic acidosis].

  b. **Urinalysis** indicates elevated glucose and ketone levels; this test allows rapid diagnosis of the condition.

  c. **Serum potassium levels** are initially increased because of intracellular shifts secondary to acidosis; later, serum potassium levels decrease as acidosis is corrected.

4. Treatment

    a. If **vascular collapse** is evident, **insulin** should be given intravenously at an initial dose of 0.1 U/kg of regular insulin.

        (1) This dose should be followed by an infusion of 0.1 U/kg/h, with frequent glucose monitoring and titration of the infusion.

        (2) Treatment with intermediate-acting insulin is resumed after acute hyperglycemia and acidosis are corrected.

    b. Because a 3- to 5-L fluid deficit usually exists, **fluids** should be given.

        (1) One liter of normal saline (0.9%) per hour for 2 hours is given, followed by a decreased rate to complete the rehydration process.

        (2) When serum glucose levels decrease to between 200 and 300 mg/dl, a **5% or 10% solution of glucose** is added to the infusion to prevent hypoglycemia.

    c. When **levels of potassium** decrease toward normal, 20 to 40 mmol/h should be infused intravenously; HCO_3 is given only if pH falls below 7.1.

C. Hyperosmolar nonketotic coma

    1. General characteristics

        a. This condition **occurs primarily in elderly patients who have NIDDM.**

        b. **Hyperglycemia** occurs secondary to stress of illness or increased glucose ingestion over days to weeks → osmotic diuresis → dehydration (if patient is unable to maintain adequate oral fluid intake) → progressive decline in mental status.

        c. **Ketoacidosis** does not occur because NIDDM patients have sufficient insulin to inhibit ketogenesis.

    2. Clinical features

        a. **Signs of dehydration** (tachycardia, dry mucous membranes, poor skin turgor, and postural hypotension) are evident.

        b. Patients exhibit **cloudy sensorium** that may progress to coma.

        c. **Seizures** can occur.

    3. Laboratory findings

        a. **Serum analysis** indicates glucose levels often reaching 1000 mg/dl, which produce elevated serum osmolality and increased urea: creatinine ratio (indicative of dehydration).

        b. **Mild metabolic acidosis** secondary to decreased renal excretion of organic acids as well as from starvation ketosis may be present.

    4. Treatment

        a. Therapy is **similar to that for DKA** (fluids, insulin, and electrolyte replacement).

        b. Because this complication is often secondary to infection, a **septic work-up** is indicated for these patients.

D. Hypoglycemic coma

    1. General characteristics

        a. Hypoglycemic coma must be rapidly **differentiated from DKA or hyperglycemic nonketotic coma.**

        b. This condition often occurs secondary to excess insulin, delayed ingestion of meals, or excess physical activity.

        c. Less commonly, it may be secondary to an insulinoma.

    2. Clinical features

        a. Sweating is important to recognize, because the DKA patient is dehydrated with dry skin.

      b. Other signs and symptoms include tachycardia, tremulousness, and palpitations secondary to adrenergic stimulation.

      c. Symptoms may then **progress to somnolence, confusion, and coma.**

  3. Laboratory findings

      a. Fingerstick blood glucose analysis provides a rapid means of hypoglycemia diagnosis.

      b. In the instance of **insulinoma,** elevated serum insulin levels are found with hypoglycemia.

      c. CT scan is effective in detecting insulinomas.

  4. Treatment

      a. Fifty milliliters of 50% glucose is given intravenously over 3 to 5 minutes, followed by a constant infusion of 5% or 10% glucose at a rate sufficient to maintain serum glucose levels > 100 mg/dl.

      b. Therapy may be required for several days, depending upon the duration of action of insulin or the oral hypoglycemic agent involved.

V. ADRENAL GLAND DYSFUNCTION

  A. Disorders affecting the adrenal cortex include Cushing's syndrome, Addison's disease, primary aldosteronism, and congenital adrenal hyperplasia; **pheochromocytoma affects the adrenal medulla.**

  B. Cushing's syndrome

    1. General characteristics

      a. Cushing's syndrome is **most commonly caused by administration of large doses of steroids** for treatment of a primary disease.

      b. If not iatrogenic, this syndrome is **most commonly caused by increased levels of pituitary ACTH,** which leads to adrenal gland hyperplasia and increased serum cortisol levels (known as Cushing's disease).

      c. Cushing's syndrome also may be caused by **adrenal adenoma or carcinoma or ectopic ACTH production from tumors** such as oat cell carcinoma of the lung.

    2. Clinical features

      a. Patients exhibit central obesity, facial plethora, buffalo hump, supraclavicular fat pads, and purple striae (linear marks) on the abdomen.

      b. Mild hypertension secondary to the vascular effects of cortisol and sodium retention may occur.

      c. Patients have **impaired glucose tolerance; 20% have overt diabetes.**

      d. Androgen excess leads to acne, hirsutism, and oligomenorrhea; however, men may complain of impotence and loss of libido.

      e. Catabolic changes occur, including muscle weakness and breakdown.

      f. Patients **bruise easily** secondary to enhanced capillary fragility.

      g. Increased bone catabolism leads to osteoporosis.

      h. Depression is not an uncommon association.

    3. Laboratory findings

      a. Diurnal variation in serum cortisol is absent.

      b. Twenty-four-hour urinary free cortisol excretion is often variable and is therefore not a useful screening test, but it may show increased cortisol excretion.

      c. Serum glucose levels are elevated, and **leukocytosis** is present (nonspecific findings).

Table 2-3

Standard Dexamethasone Suppression Test Results

Patient Type	Suppression with Low Dose	Suppression with High Dose
Normal	+	+
Adrenal tumor	−	−
Ectopic ACTH production	−	−
Cushing's disease _(pituitary)_	−	+

ACTH = adrenocorticotropic hormone.

    d. The **overnight dexamethasone suppression test** is a useful screening tool.

        (1) When taken at night, dexamethasone normally suppresses ACTH secretion and hence decreases the morning serum cortisol level.

        (2) Morning cortisol levels of >5 to 10 $\mu g/dl$ suggest Cushing's syndrome, but further testing is required because false-positive results can occur.

    e. The **standard dexamethasone suppression test** analyzes the response to low-dose and high-dose dexamethasone.

        (1) Patients who have Cushing's disease (adrenal hyperplasia) will exhibit suppressed adrenal function with high-dose dexamethasone only.

        (2) Patients who have adrenal tumors or ectopic ACTH production will not respond to dexamethasone suppression (Table 2-3).

    f. **CT scan of the adrenal glands** reveals adrenal hyperplasia but does not distinguish between ACTH stimulation from a pituitary source or ectopic source; **CT of the head** may reveal pituitary adenoma.

  4. Treatment

    a. Adrenal adenoma

        (1) **Surgical resection of the tumor** often results in cure.

        (2) **Postoperative cortisol replacement** is required for a few months until the remaining normal adrenal tissue resumes function.

    b. Adrenal carcinoma

        (1) **Surgical resection** is often not possible; once the diagnosis is made, surgery is associated with a poor outcome.

        (2) **Symptomatic relief** may be achieved through the use of adrenal steroid production-inhibiting drugs (mitotane, metyrapone, aminoglutethimide).

    c. Ectopic ACTH-producing tumors

        (1) The **tumor** itself is **usually of greater clinical significance than the resulting cortisol excess.**

        (2) These tumors are **usually not resectable.**

    d. Cushing's disease

        (1) **Transsphenoidal pituitary surgery** is the treatment of choice, with success rates approaching 95%.

        (2) **Pituitary irradiation** is effective in children but not as effective in adults.

        (3) **Bilateral adrenalectomy** results in the need for permanent steroid replacement and may result in rapid growth of the pituitary adenoma due to the removal of the negative feedback stimulus (Nelson's syndrome).

C. Addison's disease

  1. General characteristics

    a. Addison's disease is an **adrenocortical insufficiency** most commonly caused by an idiopathic atrophy of the adrenal cortex, which is believed to be autoimmune related.

b. **Tuberculosis, bilateral adrenalectomy,** or **adrenal suppression following steroid therapy** are potential causes of Addison's disease.

c. A less common cause is **hypopituitarism** (i.e., secondary adrenal insufficiency).

2. Clinical features

a. **Cortisol deficiency–related symptoms** such as weakness, fatigue, anorexia, and weight loss are seen in virtually all affected patients.

(1) **Skin hyperpigmentation** occurs secondary to increased melanocyte-stimulating hormone (MSH); increased MSH is caused by an increase in ACTH due to lack of negative feedback stimulus from cortisol.

(2) **Orthostatic hypotension** results from a loss of cortisol's pressor effects on the vasculature.

(3) **Hypoglycemia** occurs because cortisol has anti-insulin effects on glucose homeostasis.

b. **Aldosterone deficiency–related symptoms** include **hyponatremia** due to lack of aldosterone-mediated sodium retention at the distal tubule; **hyperkalemia** occurs in association with the hyponatremia and can lead to potentially fatal cardiac arrhythmias.

c. **Adrenal crisis** is an acute, potentially fatal exacerbation of adrenal insufficiency that presents with fever, vomiting, decreased sensorium, abdominal tenderness, and vascular collapse.

3. Laboratory findings

a. **Serum analysis** indicates hyperkalemia, hyponatremia, hypoglycemia, increased eosinophil count (cortisol lowers peripheral eosinophil count), and decreased cortisol and aldosterone levels.

b. **Chest radiographic studies** may reveal a small heart.

c. **Definitive diagnosis** relies on ACTH testing.

(1) If twenty-five to forty units of ACTH infused over several hours fail to induce a significant increase in serum cortisol and urinary corticoid levels, primary adrenal insufficiency is indicated.

(2) In secondary adrenal insufficiency, the response to ACTH stimulation occurs in 3 or more days.

d. **Electrocardiogram (EKG)** shows characteristic changes of hyperkalemia, including high-peaked T waves, prolonged PR interval, heart block, and atrial asystole.

4. Treatment

a. **Glucocorticoid replacement,** usually 20 mg each morning and 10 mg each evening, is required; increased dosages are required during stressful periods (e.g., surgery or illness).

b. **Mineralocorticoid replacement** (fludrocortisone, 0.05–0.2 mg/d) is required in patients who have persistent hyponatremia, hyperkalemia, and hypotension.

c. **Adrenal crisis** is treated with 100 mg of cortisol infused over 5 to 10 minutes, followed by approximately 300 mg over the next 24 hours.

(1) **Intravenous saline** is also required to replenish lost electrolytes and volume.

(2) **Mineralocorticoids** may be necessary if hypotension and dehydration persist.

D. Primary aldosteronism

1. General characteristics

a. Primary aldosteronism is characterized by **autonomous production of aldosterone by the adrenal gland.**

b. The disease is **most commonly caused by a benign adrenal adenoma,** but can also occur secondary to bilateral adrenal hyperplasia.

c. **Autonomous aldosterone production** by the adrenal gland causes increased sodium retention in exchange for potassium and hydrogen excretion at the distal tubule.

2. Clinical features

a. **Hypertension** occurs as a result of volume expansion secondary to sodium retention.

b. **Edema** does not typically occur because a new steady state is achieved once the retained excess sodium begins to spill over into the renal filtrate.

c. **Potassium loss** may produce muscle weakness, tetany, paresthesias, and dilute urine (due to hypokalemic-induced nephropathy, which impairs the kidney's ability to concentrate urine).

d. **Metabolic alkalosis** occurs secondary to renal hydrogen ion loss.

3. Laboratory findings

a. **Hypokalemia** may be detected.

b. **Plasma levels of aldosterone that remain elevated despite sodium loading** (saline infusion) **indicate hyperaldosteronism** but do not differentiate between primary and secondary (due to increased renin activity) aldosteronism.

c. **Plasma renin activity** is **decreased in primary aldosteronism,** but **increased in the secondary form;** the **combination** of elevated aldosterone and reduced renin activity **confirms** the **diagnosis** of primary aldosteronism.

d. The **biochemical changes** are more pronounced if they are caused by an adenoma versus adrenal hyperplasia.

e. **CT scan** may enable visualization of the adenoma.

4. Treatment

a. **For adenoma,** patients respond best to **surgical removal.**

b. **For hyperplasia,** patients respond best to medical treatment, specifically **spironolactone** (a potassium-sparing diuretic that inhibits aldosterone's effects on the distal nephron).

E. Congenital adrenal hyperplasia (CAH)

1. General characteristics

a. CAH is caused by a **congenital lack of the enzyme** necessary **for cortisol synthesis.**

b. The enzyme deficiency causes **ACTH levels** to **increase,** which in turn stimulates the adrenal gland to produce excess steroids not affected by the enzyme deficiency (i.e., androgens); this leads to adrenal hyperplasia.

c. **Cortisol deficiency** is usually minimal and therefore not clinically apparent.

d. The most common enzyme deficiency is **21-hydroxylase.**

(1) The deficiency may be mild, leading only to virilization.

(2) If deficiency is severe, mineralocorticoid production (salt-losing form) is impaired.

2. Clinical features

a. **Androgen excess** produces ambiguous genitalia in the female fetus (female pseudohermaphroditism) and macrogenitosomia in the male fetus.

b. **Androgen excess** may not manifest until **later in childhood,** resulting in virilization and amenorrhea in females and precocious puberty in males.

c. **Mineralocorticoid deficiency** leads to hyperkalemia, hyponatremia, dehydration, and hypotension.

3. Laboratory findings
   a. Urinary 17-ketosteroids and **pregnanetriol levels** are elevated.
   b. Serum **testosterone, androstenedione,** and **17-hydroxyprogesterone** (cortisol precursor) **levels** are elevated.

4. Treatment
   a. **Cortisol administration** suppresses ACTH-mediated adrenal hyperplasia.
   b. **Mineralocorticoid replacement** (fludrocortisone) is prescribed for the salt-losing form.
   c. **Surgical reconstruction of external genitalia** may be performed.

F. Pheochromocytoma

1. General characteristics
   a. Pheochromocytoma is a **catecholamine-producing adrenal tumor.**
   b. This tumor is a rare cause of hypertension.
   c. Pheochromocytoma **occurs within families,** such as part of MEN type II syndrome (pheochromocytoma, hyperparathyroidism, and medullary carcinoma of the thyroid gland); it is also associated with neurofibromatosis.
   d. Pheochromocytoma is **usually not malignant.**

2. Clinical features
   a. **Signs and symptoms** include episodic hypertension, headache, sweating, palpitations, and nervousness occurring with abdominal palpation or exercise.
   b. **Weight loss** and **hyperglycemia** may also occur.

3. Laboratory findings
   a. **Analysis of urinary catecholamine and vanillylmandelic acid levels** is most useful in making the diagnosis.
   b. **Serum catecholamine concentrations** are highly variable and therefore less useful diagnostically.
   c. **Clonidine suppression test** is useful in diagnosing patients with mildly elevated catecholamines; following clonidine administration, the plasma level of norepinephrine remains elevated in patients who have pheochromocytoma.
   d. **CT scan** detects the majority of these tumors.

4. **Treatment.** Because of the dangers of catecholamine excess, **pheochromocytomas should be removed surgically.** Patients should first receive a catecholamine-receptor blocking agent (propranolol) to prevent catecholamine crisis during surgery.

VI. FEMALE REPRODUCTIVE DISORDERS

A. Reproductive disorders that have an **endocrinologic basis** include primary amenorrhea, secondary amenorrhea, and androgen excess syndromes.

B. Primary amenorrhea

1. General characteristics
   a. Primary amenorrhea is defined as the **absence of menarche after 16 years of age** (i.e., patient has never had a menstrual period).
   b. **Gonadal causes** include gonadal dysgenesis (Turner's syndrome), testicular feminization syndrome (androgen resistance), and resistant ovary syndrome (rare).
   c. **Extragonadal causes** include hypogonadotropic hypogonadism, CAH (see adrenal gland dysfunction, V), and physical abnormalities.

2. Turner's syndrome
   a. General characteristics

(1) Turner's syndrome is the **most common cause of primary amenorrhea.**

(2) Individuals who have this syndrome have a **45X chromosomal arrangement.**

(3) Turner's syndrome is **not familial** and is **not correlated with advanced maternal age.**

(4) Primary amenorrhea in Turner's syndrome is caused by **failure of ovarian development → no estrogen → increased FSH/LH** (due to absence of negative feedback).

b. **Clinical features**

(1) Persons who have Turner's syndrome are of **short stature,** between 4- and 5-feet tall.

(2) Individuals have a **short, webbed neck, epicanthal folds, low-set ears,** and **widely spaced nipples.**

(3) **Renal and cardiac abnormalities** may also occur.

(4) **Estrogen deficiency** leads to **absence of development of secondary sexual characteristics** (e.g., breast, pubic, and axillary hair); therefore, these patients often present in adolescence.

c. **Laboratory findings**

(1) **Serum FSH/LH levels** are **elevated; estrogen** is **absent.**

(2) **Chromosomal analysis** reveals **45X** (most commonly), **mosaic 46XX/45X, or mosaic 46XY/45X.**

d. **Treatment**

(1) Secondary sexual characteristics develop with **estrogen therapy.**

(2) If estrogen is given cyclically with progesterone (e.g., oral contraceptives), **menstrual cycles** will ensue.

(3) **Fertility** is impossible because ovaries are nonfunctioning.

(4) **Streak gonads** associated with the 46XY/45X mosaic chromosomal arrangement must be removed because of the increased incidence of gonadoblastoma in this population; **karyotyping** is therefore necessary.

3. **Testicular feminization syndrome (androgen resistance)**

a. **General characteristics**

(1) Individuals are **46XY** but have **female external genitalia.**

(2) Peripheral tissues are resistant to androgens; therefore, male genitalia fail to develop.

(3) Presence of **Y chromosome** leads to production of müllerian duct inhibitory factor, which exerts its normal effect of inhibiting the development of internal female reproductive organs.

(4) These individuals are **often raised as girls** and present most often at adolescence with the complaint of primary amenorrhea.

b. **Clinical features**

(1) Individuals are **phenotypic females** and have a **vagina** that ends in a blind pouch.

(2) **Hypoplastic male ducts and testes** are found in the abdomen, inguinal canal, or labia majora.

(3) **Normal breast development** occurs at puberty because of the action of endogenous estrogens.

c. **Laboratory findings.** Pelvic ultrasound easily reveals the anatomic abnormalities.

d. **Treatment**

(1) Because the **testes** may become malignant, **removal** is necessary.

(2) **Estrogen therapy** maintains secondary sexual characteristics, but menses and fertility are not possible due to lack of female reproductive organs.

4. Hypogonadotropic hypogonadism
   a. General characteristics
      (1) Hypogonadotropic hypogonadism may be associated with **panhypopituitarism** that occurs before the onset of menses, and therefore, patients will have been seen previously with other symptoms of **hypopituitarism.**
      (2) The condition is also caused by isolated gonadotropin releasing hormone (Gn-RH) deficiency; **Gn-RH deficiency** most commonly occurs secondary to stress such as infection, death of a loved one, excessive exercise and dieting, and anorexia nervosa.
      (3) The condition may be caused by a **prolactinoma;** the patient presents with **amenorrhea** and **galactorrhea** (see disorders of the pituitary gland, I B 2 b).
   b. Laboratory findings
      (1) **Low circulating estrogens and FSH/LH levels** are found.
      (2) Patients show **no response to the progesterone withdrawal test.**
         (a) In the test, progesterone is administered for 5 days; menstrual bleeding should occur after progesterone is withdrawn if sufficient estrogens are present to induce uterine proliferation.
         (b) Patients show a **positive response** (i.e., menses) **to estrogen priming followed by progesterone withdrawal;** this result is indicative of functioning end organs.
   c. Treatment
      (1) Condition may resolve if the **stressful event** is **reversed.**
      (2) **Estrogen therapy** induces menses and maintains secondary sexual characteristics.
      (3) **Cyclic estrogen–progesterone therapy** induces menses, but suppresses ovulation.
      (4) **Gonadotropin hormone** can be administered if pregnancy is desired.

5. Physical abnormalities
   a. Physical abnormalities that can lead to primary amenorrhea include:
      (1) **Labial agglutination** (fusion); this condition, often associated with ambiguous genitalia, may be seen in disorders such as CAH.
      (2) **Congenital defects of the vagina** or **imperforate hymen**
      (3) **Transverse vaginal septae**
   b. These patients are seen with **cyclic abdominal pain** because menstrual outflow is impeded.

C. Secondary amenorrhea

   1. Secondary amenorrhea is defined as the **cessation of menses for 3 to 6 months** in a normally menstruating woman.

   2. Causes of secondary amenorrhea include:
      a. **Pregnancy followed by hypothalamic** (functional) **amenorrhea,** in which Gn-RH levels are decreased, often secondary to psychological stress (most common cause of secondary amenorrhea)
      b. **Anorexia nervosa and excessive exercise** (e.g., marathon runners)
      c. **Postpill amenorrhea,** defined as the absence of menses 6 months after discontinuation of oral contraceptives (uncommon)
      d. **Primary ovarian failure** (early menopause), which **occurs before 40 years of age** secondary to a decline in ovarian function (caused by autoantibodies) and leads to decreased estrogen and increased gonadotropin levels
      e. **Granulosa–theca ovarian tumor,** which may inhibit menses through excess production of estrogens; less common

D. Androgen excess syndromes: polycystic ovary disease

1. Androgen excess syndromes include polycystic ovary syndrome, androgen-producing ovarian tumors, adrenal tumors, and CAH. Only polycystic ovary disease is discussed here because the other clinical entities occur relatively infrequently.

2. General characteristics
   a. Polycystic ovary disease causes **chronic anovulation** associated with androgen excess and obesity.
   b. Approximately **5% of reproductive-age women** have polycystic ovary disease.
   c. Ovary produces **excess androstenedione** (androgenic steroid), which is converted in the periphery to estrone.
   d. **Excess androgenic steroids** prevent follicular maturation, which leads to anovulation.
   e. **Increased levels of circulating estrone** have positive feedback on LH secretion and inhibit FSH secretion, which leads to enlarged ovaries with small follicular cysts.
   f. **Unopposed estrogens** (i.e., no ovulation and therefore no progesterone) may increase risk of endometrial cancer in this population.

3. Clinical features
   a. **Chronic anovulation** leads to infertility and menstrual irregularities such as oligomenorrhea or amenorrhea.
   b. **Oily skin, hirsutism,** and **acne** occur because of androgen excess.
   c. **Obesity** is often present.

4. Laboratory findings
   a. **LH-FSH ratio** is increased (>2), **LH level** is elevated, and **FSH level** is low to normal.
   b. **Serum testosterone** and **androstenedione levels** are elevated.
   c. **Estrone** (estrogen formed in peripheral tissues) **level** is elevated; **estradiol level** is normal.

5. Treatment
   a. Signs and symptoms of androgen excess can be alleviated with **estrogen–progestin combinations** that decrease androgen levels.
      (1) Glucocorticoids may also be used because they suppress adrenal-derived androgens.
      (2) Spironolactone, a potassium-sparing diuretic, also decreases androgen synthesis and hair follicle stimulation.
   b. If fertility is desired, **clomiphene** can be used; clomiphene blocks negative feedback of estrogen, increasing FSH and LH levels and thereby stimulating follicular growth and ovulation.

E. Diagnostic evaluation of the amenorrheic patient

1. Pregnancy test [serum β-human chorionic gonadotropin (HCG) level] should be performed before any other diagnostic procedure, even in primary amenorrhea.

2. Progesterone withdrawal test (10 mg medroxyprogesterone daily for 5 days) is the second diagnostic test for amenorrhea.
   a. **Withdrawal bleeding** suggests that sufficient estrogen production is present for uterine proliferation and that the lack of menses is due to anovulation.
   b. If withdrawal bleeding does not occur, proceed to Diagnostic Step 3.

3. Estrogen–progesterone withdrawal test is the third diagnostic test for amenorrhea (Premarin [a conjugated estrogen] 1.25 mg for 21 days followed by the progesterone withdrawal test).

    a. This test **induces menses if the endometrium and outflow tract are normal** (physical abnormalities should be readily detectable by physical examination before diagnostic evaluation).

    b. If **no bleeding** occurs, the patient should be referred to a gynecologist for further investigation.

    c. **Bleeding** suggests either ovarian dysfunction or hypothalamic–pituitary disease, which can be distinguished by Diagnostic Step 4.

4. **Measurement of serum gonadotropin levels** is the fourth diagnostic test for amenorrhea.

    a. **Elevated levels** indicate ovarian disease.

    b. **Low gonadotropin level** indicates hypothalamic-pituitary dysfunction, which may be secondary to a prolactinoma; hence, prolactin levels should also be measured (especially if galactorrhea is also present).

    c. **Elevated LH-FSH ratio** suggests polycystic ovary disease.

VII. MALE REPRODUCTIVE DISORDERS

A. The major reproductive disorders in men include hypogonadism and gynecomastia.

B. Hypogonadism

    1. **General characteristics**

        a. Hypogonadism results in **inadequate testosterone and sperm production.**

        b. Hypogonadotropic hypogonadism indicates that the testes lack stimulation from a diseased hypothalamic–pituitary axis; this condition may manifest as delayed puberty.

        c. Hypergonadotropic hypogonadism indicates a disorder within the testes themselves, and that negative feedback on the hypothalamic–pituitary axis is absent.

            1. **Klinefelter's syndrome** (47XXY karyotype) results in congenital testicular damage, eunuchoidism, and gynecomastia.

            2. **Testicular agenesis** results in failure of pubertal development and absence of testes (although testes were present during embryogenesis, because these individuals have male genitalia).

            3. **Mumps orchitis** affects both testes and results in hypergonadotropic hypogonadism.

    2. **Treatment**

        a. **Depo-Testosterone** is necessary for full virilization.

        b. Infertility cannot be corrected in primary testicular damage; however, **Gn-RH** is effective for individuals who have hypogonadotropic hypogonadism.

C. Gynecomastia

    1. Gynecomastia is a group of disorders that cause **male breast development** and may involve estrogen excess, decreased levels of androgens, or both.

    2. Gynecomastia in **newborns** is common and subsides spontaneously in weeks to months.

    3. Two thirds of normal boys develop some degree of gynecomastia during puberty that subsides in 1 to 2 years; therefore, no diagnostic studies are indicated.

    4. **Hypogonadism** may be associated with gynecomastia.

    5. **Liver diseases** such as cirrhosis lead to increased estrogen and breast development (results of liver function tests are abnormal).

6. Tumors such as testicular choriocarcinoma (which secretes chorionic gonadotropin) cause testicular estrogen production, which leads to gynecomastia (diagnosis should be suspected from elevated β-HCG level).

7. Gynecomastia can be **drug-induced,** as from marijuana, phenothiazines, tricyclic antidepressants, digitalis, and cimetidine.

VIII. DISORDERS OF BONE METABOLISM

A. Osteoporosis

1. General characteristics
  a. Osteoporosis is characterized by **decreased bone volume;** bone structure is normal.
  b. This disease is **familial** and predominates in **Caucasian women.** *Asian*
  c. Calcium deficiency can increase bone resorption and osteoporosis.
  d. Estrogen has a protective effect on bone; therefore, osteoporosis is more common in postmenopausal women.
  e. Osteoporosis may be **secondary to malabsorption syndromes, steroid therapy,** or **multiple myeloma.**

2. Clinical features
  a. Vertebral compression fractures in the lower thoracic and lumbar vertebrae occur, the initial symptoms of which may be **acute back pain.**
  b. Femur fractures (at the neck) are also common.

3. Laboratory findings
  a. Radiography reveals decreased bone density if bone loss is more than 30%.
  b. Wedge-shaped deformities are characteristic of vertebral compression fractures (Figure 2-1).

4. Treatment
  a. Estrogen replacement therapy (ERT) in the postmenopausal woman can prevent or slow the rate of osteoporosis development; ERT is contraindicated in women who are at high risk for endometrial or breast cancer.
  b. Calcium supplementation (e.g., Fosamax) is essential to maintain bone mass (1500 mg/day) and prevent or slow osteoporosis.
  c. Weight-bearing exercise and an **active lifestyle** may help prevent osteoporosis.

B. Osteomalacia

1. General characteristics
  a. Osteomalacia is a disease of **inadequate mineralization of bone matrix.**
  b. Osteomalacia is caused by **vitamin D deficiency** (vitamin D is necessary for normal calcium metabolism, and deficiency of this vitamin causes **rickets** in children); vitamin D deficiency is now uncommon in the United States.
  c. Liver and renal diseases can impair vitamin D metabolism and hence lead to decreased bone mineralization.
  d. GI disorders that impair absorption interfere with vitamin D absorption and normal calcium metabolism.

2. Clinical features
  a. Pain and tenderness are felt in the spine, ribs, and lower extremities.
  b. Proximal muscle weakness results in a **waddling gait.**
  c. Lower extremities are **bowed** and **prone to fractures.**

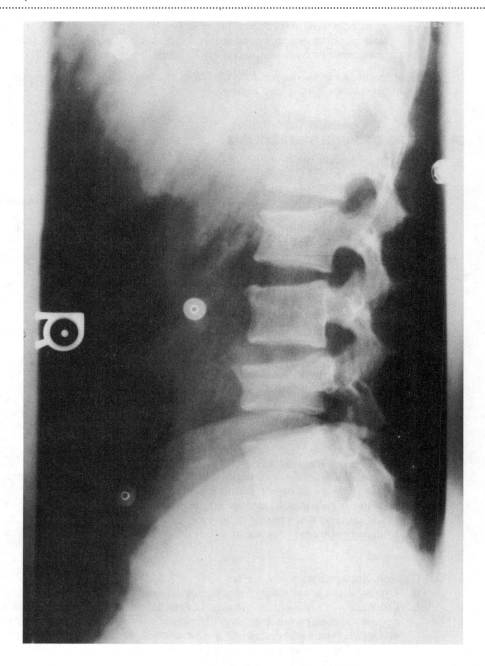

Figure 2-1.   Classic appearance of a vertebral wedge-shaped deformity associated with vertebral compression fracture in a patient with severe osteoporosis.

3. Laboratory findings

    a. **Radiography** reveals decreased bone density and coarsened trabecular pattern.

    b. **Serum analysis** indicates low serum phosphate and calcium levels and elevated alkaline phosphatase level.

4. Treatment

    a. Therapy should treat the primary disorder affecting the abnormal calcium metabolism.

    b. **Vitamin D** benefits individuals who have a lack or impairment in metabolism of the vitamin.

    c. **Supplemental calcium** is **of little benefit** because the disorder is not caused by calcium deficiency; however, during bone reformation, calcium supplements may be necessary.

3

Renal, Fluid, and Electrolyte Disorders

I. RENAL FAILURE

A. Acute renal failure (ARF)

1. General characteristics

a. ARF is an **abrupt reduction in kidney function** that results from a variety of causes (Table 3-1).

b. ARF is **usually reversible.**

2. Clinical features

a. **Signs and symptoms** of ARF depend on etiology.

b. **Oliguria** (<400 ml/day) **or anuria** (<100 ml/day) may be present; however, patients may still produce urine and have ARF if acute azotemia is present.

c. Patient may be **edematous and hypertensive** if the cause is renal.

d. **Orthostatic hypotension, tachycardia, and dry mucous membranes** are indicative of prerenal causes.

e. **Tympanic lower abdomen** may be present if bladder outflow is obstructed (e.g., Foley catheter obstruction).

3. Laboratory findings

a. **Serum urea and creatinine levels are elevated;** if the ratio of blood urea nitrogen to creatinine is more than 20:1, then the cause of the ARF is likely prerenal.

b. In prerenal ARF, **fractional excretion of sodium** (FE_{Na}) < 1% = ($urine_{Na}$/$plasma_{Na}$) ($plasma_{Cr}$/$urine_{Cr}$),provided that the patient has not recently used loop diuretics.

c. $Urine_{Osm}$ more than 400 mOsm/kg **and** $urine_{Na}$ less than 20 mmol/L are laboratory results usually **consistent with prerenal causes.**

d. **Urinary sediment** (urinalysis) reveals granular casts, which indicate acute tubular necrosis or nephrotoxins.

(1) **White blood cells** and/or white blood cell casts suggest interstitial nephritis (as seen with drug allergies or infections).

(2) **Red blood cells** (RBCs) (or more specifically, RBC casts) suggest glomerulonephritis.

e. If urinalysis indicates renal parenchymal disease, a **renal biopsy** may be indicated to differentiate conditions that may respond to steroid or immunosuppressive therapy.

4. Treatment

a. **Treatment depends on the cause** of ARF.

b. **Hypovolemia** should be treated with rehydration.

46

Table 3-1
Causes of Acute Renal Failure

Prerenal	Postrenal	Renal
Hypoperfusion secondary to hypovolemia, blood loss, dehydration *shock* Maldistribution, as in sepsis or liver disease, low cardiac output	Urinary tract obstruction: renal ultrasound can quickly diagnose acute obstruction	Interstitial disease (interstitial nephritis or acute tubular necrosis)* Glomerular disease Renovascular disease

* Interstitial nephritis may be associated with the use of antibiotics or non-steroidal anti-inflammatory drugs; acute tubular necrosis may be secondary to myoglobinemia, uric acidemia (large tumor load), cytotoxic chemotherapy, the use of radiocontrast material, or aminogycosides.

    c. **Obstruction** may require catheterization and removal if obstruction (e.g., calculi) has been present for more than 5 days.

    d. Appropriate **therapy for renal disease** should be initiated, if necessary (see glomerulonephropathies, II B).

    e. Established **renal failure requires dialysis** until patient enters the recovery phase.

B. Chronic renal failure/end-stage renal disease

    1. General characteristics

        a. **Signs and symptoms** of chronic renal failure do not occur until approximately 90% of normal renal function is lost.

        b. Chronic renal failure is defined as **renal function between 5% and 25% of normal function.**

            (1) This condition usually does not require dialysis and is asymptomatic.

            (2) Patients may require erythropoietin, phosphate binders, and vitamin D.

        c. **End-stage renal disease** is defined as less than 5% of normal renal function; patients require dialysis, erythropoietin, and hormone replacement.

        d. **Causes** of chronic renal failure include chronic glomerulonephritis, chronic reflux nephropathy, chronic pyelonephritis, diabetes mellitus, malignant hypertension or bilateral renovascular disease (essential hypertension rarely leads to end-stage renal disease), and polycystic kidney disease.

    2. Clinical features

        a. If untreated, patients may become **edematous** and **hypertensive.**

        b. **Tachypnea** may be present if metabolic acidosis has occurred.

        c. **Hyperkalemia** may lead to a catastrophic cardiac event (i.e., asystole).

        d. **Osteodystrophy** occurs secondary to decreased renal formation of 1,25-dihydroxyvitamin D and increased levels of parathyroid hormone secondary to poor phosphate excretion.

        e. **Uremic toxin-associated signs and symptoms** include anorexia, nausea, vomiting, and malaise.

        f. **Conditions associated with uremic toxemia** include:

            (1) Metabolic encephalopathy

            (2) Pleuropericarditis

            (3) Volume-dependent hypertension and pulmonary edema

            (4) Peripheral neuropathy

            (5) Pruritus

            (6) Volume-independent hypertension

            (7) Platelet dysfunction

3. Laboratory findings
   a. **Normochromic, normocytic anemia** may be present.
   b. Patients are **hyperkalemic.**
   c. **Anion-gap acidosis** may be present.
   d. **Serum phosphate levels** are elevated, and **serum calcium levels** are decreased.
   e. **Serum urea and creatinine levels** are elevated.

4. Treatment
   a. Treatment for end-stage renal disease involves **dialysis** until a successful kidney transplantation can be performed.
   b. **Phosphate binders** may decrease intestinal phosphate absorption.
   c. Patients should receive **erythropoietin therapy** and **calcium** and **vitamin D** supplements.

II. ABNORMAL URINALYSIS AND GLOMERULONEPHROPATHY

A. Abnormal urinalysis

1. **General characteristics**
   a. Abnormal urinalysis indicative of renal pathology involves either **proteinuria** or some forms of **hematuria** (discussed in parts 2 and 3 of this section), or both.
   b. Understanding the significance of an **active urinary sediment** can aid the diagnosis of glomerulonephropathy.

2. **Proteinuria**
   a. A **24-hour urine collection** must be obtained if proteinuria is detected on initial urinalysis, and the cause is unclear.
   b. Proteinuria more than 2.0 g/day is **usually due to a glomerulonephropathy** (i.e., glomerular disease).
   c. Proteinuria greater than 3.5 g/day is **indicative of nephrotic syndrome** (see glomerulonephropathies, II B); this degree of proteinuria is **not** seen in interstitial or tubular disease.
   d. Proteinuria less than 2.0 g/day is **associated with interstitial or tubular disease** (e.g., acute tubular necrosis, interstitial nephritis, pyelonephritis), but **does not** exclude glomerulonephropathy.
   e. **Malignant hypertension** may be associated with glomerular range proteinuria (>2.0 g/day), but **chronic mild or moderate essential hypertension** is typically associated with proteinuria of less than 1.0 g/day.
   f. **Complications of excessive renal protein loss** include edema secondary to decreased oncotic pressure, hyperlipidemia, hypercoagulable state, hypogammaglobulinemia, and vitamin D deficiency (vitamin D is bound to filtered protein and is therefore lost).

3. **Hematuria**
   a. **General characteristics**
      (1) Hematuria may arise anywhere along the genitourinary tract from the kidneys to the urethra.
      (2) **Glomerular hematuria** occurs when a glomerulonephritis is present (for which there are several causes).
      (3) **Non-glomerular origin hematuria** may be the result of trauma, stones, tumors, or infection involving any part of the genitourinary tract.
   b. Glomerular hematuria can be distinguished from non-glomerular hematuria by the following:
      (1) **Presence of RBC casts** is pathognomonic for acute glomerulonephritis; however, RBC casts are not always present.

(2) Glomerular range proteinuria (>2.0 g/day) **with hematuria** indicates a glomerular origin.

(3) Crenated RBCs in the urine are a product of glomerular disease, whereas **normal RBCs** arise from non-glomerular hemorrhage.

B. Glomerulonephropathies

1. General characteristics

  a. Glomerulonephropathies (GN) may be **diffuse** (involving all glomeruli), **focal** (involving only some of the glomeruli), or **segmental** (involving a portion of each individual glomerulus).

  b. The condition may be **primary** (disease process is localized to the kidney) or **secondary** to an underlying disease.

  c. GNs are divided into two main categories: **proliferative glomerulonephropathies** and **non-proliferative glomerulonephropathies.**

2. Proliferative glomerulonephropathies

  a. General characteristics

   (1) Urinalysis reveals presence of RBCs (>20 RBCs/high-powered field) and +/− RBC casts; **proteinuria** is present in variable amounts.

   (2) This condition involves a diffuse or focal proliferation of glomerular cells.

   (3) In **primary glomerulonephropathy,** disease is primary to the kidney; in **secondary glomerulonephropathy,** underlying disease produces renal damage.

   (4) Patients may present with acute or chronic symptoms of renal failure (see renal failure, I A 2).

   (5) Primary causes are commonly associated with either post-streptococcal glomerulonephritis or IgA nephropathy (Berger's disease).

  b. Post-streptococcal glomerulonephritis

   (1) This condition occurs acutely 10 to 20 days after a pharyngeal or cutaneous streptococcal infection.

   (2) Signs and symptoms include gross hematuria, proteinuria, edema, and hypertension.

   (3) Serum C3 levels are temporarily reduced (less than 8 weeks' duration).

  c. Immunoglobulin A (IgA) nephropathy

   (1) This condition is the **most common cause of glomerular origin hematuria.**

   (2) IgA nephropathy is **associated with deposits of IgA** in the renal mesangium.

   (3) Patients are seen with **recurrent, gross hematuria** immediately following upper respiratory tract or gastrointestinal tract infection (no lag of 10–20 days, as seen with the post-streptococcal infection).

   (4) Urinalysis may be normal between episodes.

   (5) The presence of **hypertension** is **associated with a poor prognosis** (i.e., patients develop end-stage renal disease).

   (6) Serum C3 levels are normal.

   (7) Linear pattern along basement membrane is detected by immunofluorescence study.

  d. Goodpasture's disease is another primary form of proliferative GN, which is also associated with pulmonary hemorrhage and involves anti-glomerular basement membrane antibodies.

  e. Secondary causes of proliferative GN include systemic lupus erythematosus (SLE), Henoch-Schönlein purpura, Wegener's granulomatosis, and polyarteritis nodosa (see Chapter 1 on rheumatic diseases).

3. Non-proliferative glomerulonephropathies

    a. Non-proliferative GNs involve disease of the glomerular basement membrane without proliferation of cells.

    b. A patient who has this condition may be initially seen with hypertension.

    c. **Urinalysis** reveals glomerular range proteinuria, few RBCs (usually <5 per high-powered field), and **no** RBC casts.

    d. Non-proliferative GNs may be primary or secondary.

    e. **Secondary causes** include general malignancy, SLE, gold and penicillamine therapy, heroin use, ureteroreflux, acquired immunodeficiency syndrome, paraproteinemia secondary to multiple myeloma or amyloid, and diabetes mellitus.

    f. Histologic type known as **minimal change disease** is common in the pediatric population, which is usually associated with both normal glomerular filtration rate and blood pressure, and has a good prognosis following steroid therapy.

    g. **Pre-eclampsia** is associated with non-proliferative glomerulonephropathy.

III. RENAL CALCULI

A. General characteristics

1. Approximately 1 in 10 persons in the United States has renal calculi.

2. Renal calculi are **twice as common in men** as compared with women and are **uncommon in children.**

3. Renal calculi are **commonly composed of calcium** (80% of all renal calculi), **magnesium ammonium sulfate** (struvite or infection stones), or, less frequently, **uric acid.**

B. Clinical features

1. **Fever** may be present.

2. Patients assume a **severe ipsilateral costovertebral angle** and report **lower back pain** and tenderness.

3. **Gross hematuria** may be present.

4. **Decreased urine output** may be noted.

C. Laboratory findings

1. Laboratory results **vary with stone type.**

2. Urine should be sent for **culture and sensitivity** to rule out struvite stones and pyelonephritis.

3. **Urinalysis** should be performed to assess for the presence of stone-specific crystals.

4. **A 24-hour urine collection** is used to identify the presence of excess levels of stone-forming substrates such as calcium or uric acid.

5. **Serum electrolytes,** including calcium, uric acid, and phosphate **should be measured,** because elevated levels of these substances may reveal the composition of the stone.

6. **Intravenous pyelogram** is often diagnostic of the presence of renal calculi.

7. **Plain radiographic studies** may reveal the location of the stone if it is radiopaque (uric acid stones are radiolucent; calcium stones are radiopaque).

8. **Renal ultrasound** or **computed tomographic scan** is also effective in identifying stones.

D. Treatment

1. Patients should be given **adequate pain medication over 3 to 5 days,** during which time they are likely to pass the stone.

2. **Fluid intake** is encouraged, and **diuretics** (particularly thiazides, which lower urinary calcium) may be of some benefit in preventing recurrence.

3. **Allopurinol** is useful in treating patients who have uric acid stones.

4. **Orthophosphate** can be used in patients who have hypercalciuria and calcium stones to decrease the absorption of dietary calcium.

IV. RENOVASCULAR DISEASE

A. General characteristics

1. **Renal artery stenosis** is the most common cause of secondary hypertension (accounts for 5% of all persons who have hypertensive disease), which is usually secondary to atherosclerotic narrowing of the renal artery.

2. **Secondary hypertension** is more common in younger patients, elderly patients who have new onset of hypertension, and persons who have malignant hypertension.

3. Secondary hypertension results in **stimulation of the renin-angiotensin-aldosterone system.**

4. **Renovascular disease** may be less commonly due to fibromuscular disease (seen in young women), localized aneurysms, and space-occupying lesions of the kidney such as cysts or tumors.

B. Clinical features

1. **Patients are hypertensive** (hypertension may be in the malignant hypertensive range, with diastolic >120 mm Hg).

2. **Evidence of peripheral vascular disease** may be present along with a **history of intermittent claudication.**

3. **Midabdominal bruit** may be present.

4. Patients are resistant to **anti-hypertensive medications.**

5. **Muscle weakness and tetany** may occur secondary to hypokalemia.

C. Laboratory findings

1. **Hypokalemia** may be present.

2. **Captopril test results** are **positive;** that is, a significant increase in plasma renin activity is detected following administration of captopril (an angiotensin converting enzyme inhibitor).

3. **Digital subtraction renal arteriography** should be performed if the captopril test is positive in order to reveal the location of the stenosis; in contrast to bilateral arteriography, this test does not require arterial cannulation.

4. If digital subtraction is nondiagnostic, **bilateral arteriography** should then be performed.

D. Treatment

1. Surgery and **angioplasty** are **superior to medical therapy,** because the former thera-pies relieve the stenosis, thereby eliminating the cause of the hypertension as well as restoring normal blood flow to the affected kidney.

2. Angioplasty should be attempted in short lesions because it is less invasive than surgery (especially in patients who are poor surgical candidates).

V. ASSESSMENT AND DIAGNOSIS OF VOLUME AND ELECTROLYTE DISORDERS

A. General considerations

1. Assessment of volume disturbances requires a **clinical evaluation** of the patient as well as **assessment of the patient's serum sodium level** to determine the most appropriate course.

2. Dehydration indicates a decrease in the total body sodium level.

3. Serum sodium is a measure of sodium concentration and therefore indicates the body's relative need for free water.

a. If the serum sodium level is elevated, the patient needs free water in order to return the sodium concentration to normal.

b. If the serum sodium level is decreased, the patient has more free water relative to sodium.

4. Appropriate **treatment of the patient who has sodium and water imbalances** in-volves an assessment of both the serum sodium level **and** the patient's volume status.

B. Hyponatremia

1. Hyponatremia may occur:

a. With an increased total body sodium level (the patient is edematous and hence has an increased total body sodium level; however, total body water also in-creases, producing a relative hyponatremia)

b. With a decreased total body sodium level (the patient appears dehydrated and hence has a decreased total body sodium level)

c. With a normal total body sodium level (the patient appears euvolemic and hence has a normal total body sodium level but an increase in total body water, for example, syndrome of inappropriate antidiuretic hormone).

d. Secondary to pseudohyponatremia

2. The following equation determines the osmolar gap.

osmolar gap = calculated osmolarity − measured osmolarity

calculated osmolarity = 2(serum Na) + glucose(mmol/L) + urea (mmol/L)

a. The osmolar gap should be less than 10; if it is more than 10, then one of the following is true (see Table 3-2):

Table 3-2
Differential for Increased Osmolar Gap

Measured	Calculated	Cause
Normal	Low	Pseudohyponatremia secondary to abnormal lipid protein levels
High	Normal	Search for abnormal solute levels (e.g., alcohol ethylene glycol, methanol)
Low	Normal	Laboratory error

b. The **true [Na] level** can be determined by adding 3 mmol/L of Na to the serum [Na] level for every 10-mmol increase in serum glucose.

c. **Hypernatremia** can be evaluated clinically in a manner similar to that of hyponatremia (see Figures 3-1 and 3-2).

C. Hyperkalemia and hypokalemia

1. General considerations

   a. **Chronic changes in potassium levels** occur as a result of renal potassium handling.

   b. **Acute changes in potassium levels** are governed by:

      (1) **Increased sympathetic drive** (causing increased cellular uptake of potassium, which leads to hypokalemia)

      (2) **Insulin** (increased cellular uptake also causes hypokalemia)

      (3) **Acidosis** (increased cellular efflux of potassium with influx of hydrogen ions, which leads to hyperkalemia)

      (4) **Alkalosis** (increased efflux of hydrogen ions and influx of potassium, which leads to hypokalemia)

2. **Assessment of hypokalemia is shown in Figure 3-3.**

3. **Hyperkalemia can be the result of:**

   a. **False hyperkalemia**

      (1) **Hemolyzed blood sample** very common, especially if it is difficult to obtain a venous blood specimen

      (2) Recheck the **potassium level**

   b. **Massive tissue injury** that can occur with hemolysis associated with chemotherapy and cell death, or burns; dialysis or diuresis with fluid replacement may be required

   c. **Type IV RTA** (see V D)

   d. **Acute or end-stage renal failure**

D. Acid–base disorders

1. General considerations

   a. Acid–base disorders can be either **metabolic** (changes in serum [bicarbonate] level) or **respiratory** (changes in $PaCO_2$ level).

   b. An increase or decrease in **hydrogen ion concentration** may occur in either metabolic or respiratory causes; these changes lead to four possible disease processes: **metabolic acidosis** (decreased serum [bicarbonate] level), **metabolic alkalosis** (increased serum [bicarbonate] level), **respiratory acidosis** (increased $PaCO_2$ level), and **respiratory alkalosis** (decreased $PaCO_2$ level).

   c. Each of these disturbances can lead to a compensatory response by the body in an attempt to maintain a normal pH.

      (1) For example, a patient who has metabolic acidosis will begin to hyperventilate in order to increase the serum pH toward its normal value (a response that occurs in a matter of hours).

      (2) A patient who has a primary respiratory condition such as respiratory acidosis (increased $PaCO_2$ level) will develop a metabolic alkalosis (increased serum [bicarbonate] level; this response, mediated by the kidneys, may require 2 to 3 days.)

   d. Determining if a patient has one primary metabolic derangement with an appropriate physiologic response as opposed to two or three primary derangements must be accomplished in order to institute appropriate therapy.

   e. The following rules should be committed to memory:

      (1) **Metabolic acidosis:** for every 1 mol/L decrease in [bicarbonate] level, the

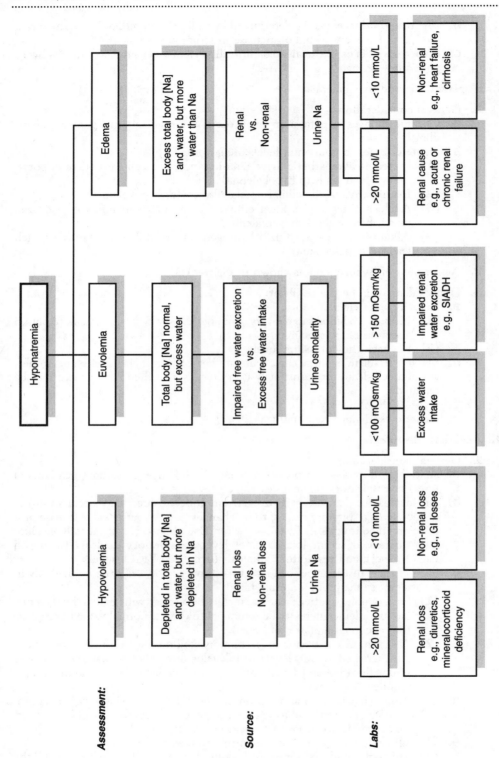

Figure 3-1.   Diagnostic approach to hyponatremia.

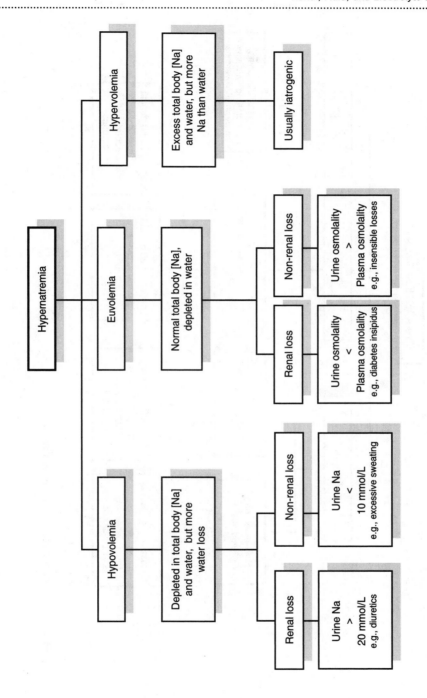

Figure 3-2. Diagnostic approach to hypernatremia.

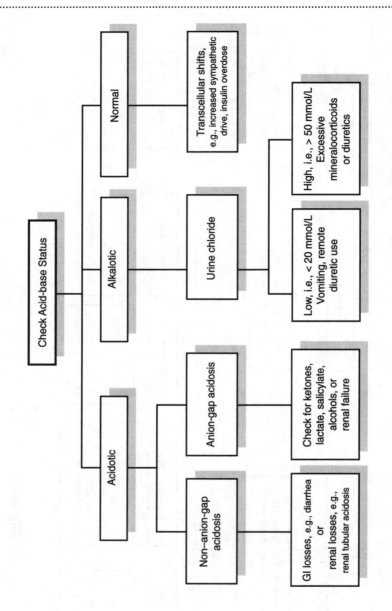

Figure 3-3.   Diagnostic approach to hypokalemia.

appropriate physiologic response is a decrease of 1.2 mm Hg in $PaCO_2$ level.

(2) **Metabolic alkalosis:** for every 1 mmol/L increase in [bicarbonate] level, the appropriate physiologic response is an increase of 0.6 mm Hg in $PaCO_2$ level.

(3) **Respiratory acidosis:** for every 1 mm Hg increase in $PaCO_2$ level, the appropriate physiologic response is an increase of 0.4 mmol/L in [bicarbonate] level.

(4) **Respiratory alkalosis:** for every 1 mm Hg decrease in $PaCO_2$ level, the appropriate physiologic response is a decrease of 0.4 mmol/L in [bicarbonate] level.

f. When calculating the appropriate physiologic response of a patient with an acid–base disturbance, allow $+/-$ 2 units.

g. Causes of metabolic acidosis and alkalosis disorders are shown in Figures 3-4 and 3-5.

Clinical Example

A patient's [HCO_3] (bicarbonate level) = 12, and his $PaCO_2$ level = 26 mm Hg. Does this patient have a metabolic acidosis with an appropriate physiologic response of respiratory alkalosis, or does the patient have a respiratory alkalosis with an appropriate physiologic response of metabolic acidosis? If the patient has a primary metabolic acidosis, the (bicarbonate level) has decreased 12 mmol/L (24 − 12 = 12). The appropriate drop in $PaCO_2$ level is 12 × 1.2 = 14.4 mm Hg; therefore, the expected $PaCO_2$ level for this patient is 40 − 14.4 = 25.6 mm Hg, which is within the accepted range of his actual $PaCO_2$ level. Therefore, the patient has a primary metabolic acidosis with an appropriate physiologic response of respiratory alkalosis.

If we were to assume that the patient's primary disturbance was a respiratory alkalosis, then the patient's physiologic response should be to decrease his [bicarbonate] level by (40 − 26)× (0.4) = 5.6. The patient's [bicarbonate] level should be 24 − 5.6 = 18.4, which it is not. Therefore, our assumption that this patient's primary acid–base disturbance was a respiratory alkalosis is incorrect.

It is important to recognize which acid–base disorder is the primary disorder and which is the appropriate physiologic response. If the patient has a primary metabolic acidosis, the cause should be ascertained and treated appropriately, after which time the patient's $PaCO_2$ level will return to normal. If the primary disorder is respiratory alkalosis, the patient is hyperventilating. The hyperventilation is chronic, because it takes 2 to 3 days for the [bicarbonate] level to increase in response. In the latter instance, one might imagine a patient on a ventilator with a setting that is too high, which results in overventilation. In this instance, the treatment is to simply readjust the ventilator settings.

If a metabolic acidosis is discovered, it must be further characterized as an anion-gap or a non–anion-gap acidosis as follows:

Anion gap = serum [Na] − serum [Cl] − serum [HCO_3]

- A normal anion gap is usually between 8 and 12 mEq/L.
- An anion gap greater than 12 mEq/L in the presence of a metabolic acidosis indicates an anion-gap metabolic acidosis.
- In the presence of an anion-gap acidosis, it is important to determine the [bicarbonate] level before the anion-gap acidosis ensues in order to detect an underlying acid–base disturbance.

Clinical Example

A patient's blood work-up reveals the following laboratory results:

[Na] = 136 mEq/L; [Cl] = 81 mEq/L; [HCO_3] = 32 mEq/L; $PaCO_2$ = 35 mm Hg

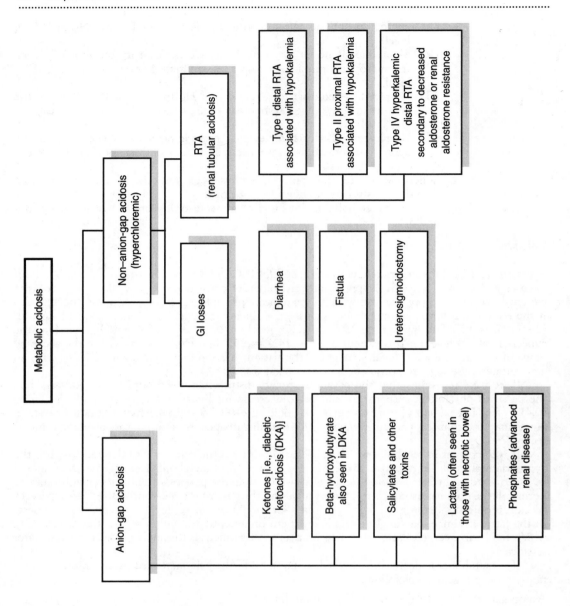

Figure 3-4. Diagnostic considerations in a patient who has metabolic acidosis.

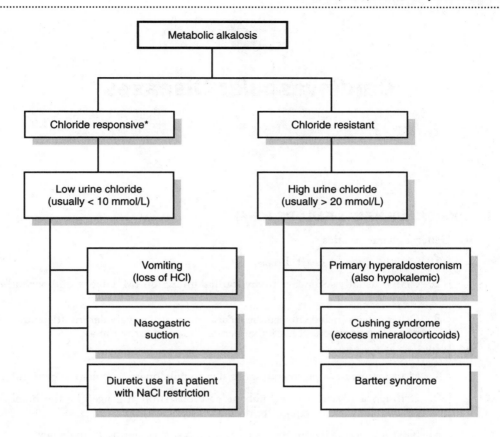

Figure 3-5. Diagnostic considerations in a patient who has metabolic alkalosis.

This patient has an elevated [bicarbonate] level; therefore, he/she may have a metabolic alkalosis. The $PaCO_2$ level should therefore be **elevated** for an appropriate physiologic response, but it is actually low. If we assume that the primary disorder is a respiratory alkalosis, then the [bicarbonate] level should be **low,** but it is elevated. Therefore, the patient has both a respiratory alkalosis and a metabolic alkalosis. Is that all?

Check the anion gap. It is 23 mEq/L (11 more than it should be). Therefore, the patient also has an anion-gap metabolic acidosis. The increase in anion gap by 11 mEq/L means that the [bicarbonate] level must have initially been 32 + 11 = 43 mEq/L before the anion-gap acidosis ensued. Therefore, this patient has a severe metabolic alkalosis that is masked by the presence of his anion-gap acidosis.

4
Cardiovascular Diseases

I. CONGESTIVE HEART FAILURE (CHF)

A. General characteristics

    1. CHF is a **sign of heart disease.**

    2. CHF is **usually secondary to myocardial infarction (MI)** due to coronary atherosclerotic disease.

    3. **Other causes** include myocarditis, cardiomyopathies, valvular insufficiency or stenosis, hypertension, constrictive pericarditis, and arrhythmias.

B. Clinical features

    1. Most frequent symptom is **dyspnea** due to pulmonary vascular congestion.

    2. **Orthopnea** (dyspnea in recumbent position) is often gauged by the number of pillows the patient requires to decrease dyspneic symptoms.

    3. **Nocturia** occurs due to increased renal blood flow during recumbency.

    4. **Lower extremity edema** occurs with right-sided heart failure.

    5. **Tachycardia** occurs as a **compensatory measure** for decreased stroke volume.

    6. **Crackles** on inspiration are caused by transudation of fluid into the alveoli.

    7. The **most reliable sign of heart failure** is the S_3 **heart sound** occurring early in diastole due to rapid filling of the left ventricle.

    8. S_4 may also occur. *CHF*

    9. **Distention of neck veins** indicating elevated **jugular venous pressures (JVP)** occurs with **right-sided failure.**

C. Laboratory findings

    1. **Laboratory results** vary, depending on the etiology of CHF.

    2. **Chest radiographic study** reveals an enlarged heart, with increased pulmonary congestion (Figure 4-1).

    3. **Echocardiogram (ECG)** is useful in determining the presence of chamber enlargement, wall motion abnormalities, decreased ejection fraction, valvular disease, and pericardial effusion.

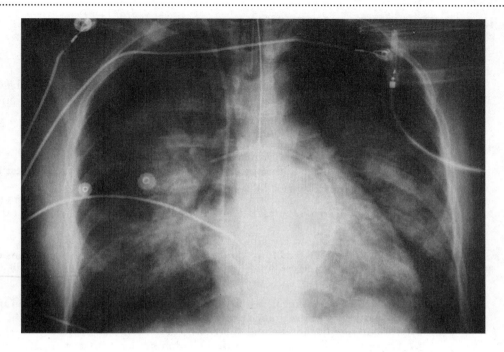

Figure 4-1.   Radiographic chest film showing acute congestive heart failure and pulmonary edema. Note the central symmetric butterfly pattern and the vascular redistribution, with increased pulmonary vascular markings at the apices of the lungs. (Reprinted with permission from Freundlich IM, Bragg DG: *A Radiologic Approach to Diseases of the Chest*, 2nd ed. Baltimore, Williams & Wilkins, p 21.)

    4. **Cardiac catheterization** is used when the etiology of the CHF must be found in order to effectively treat the underlying disease.

D. Treatment

    1. The **underlying cause** must be treated, if possible.

    2. Treatment of **pulmonary edema secondary to CHF** involves:
      a. **Oxygen** by face mask
      b. **Diuretics** (furosemide) in low initial doses, if the patient is not presently taking them   *20 mg IV*
      c. **Morphine,** if the patient is extremely anxious or is experiencing pain that increases demands on the heart
      d. **Sublingual nitroglycerin,** if the patient is experiencing **angina;** this drug is a useful adjunct to diuretic drugs in producing vasodilation, thereby reducing cardiac load
      e. **Digoxin,** which increases cardiac contractility

    3. If **oxygenation** fails to improve the patient's deteriorating condition (e.g., persistent cyanosis, obtundation), **intubation** is indicated with positive pressure ventilation.

    4. **Invasive hemodynamic monitoring** is reserved for those cases of pulmonary edema that do not resolve.

II. ISCHEMIC HEART DISEASE (IHD)

A. General characteristics

   1. The **most common cause** of IHD is **atherosclerotic disease.**

   2. **Risk factors** include increasing age, male gender, elevated serum cholesterol level, smoking, hypertension, diabetes mellitus, and family history of coronary artery disease.

B. Clinical features

   1. **Angina pectoris is caused by myocardial ischemia.**
      a. Angina pectoris is **initially precipitated by exertion and relieved by rest** but may occur at rest as IHD progresses.
      b. Patients experience **pressure or burning sensation in the chest,** with gradual onset over 2 to 3 minutes that lasts up to 20 minutes; if pain lasts longer than 30 minutes, MI is likely.
      c. **Pain** may radiate to the arm, jaw, or neck.
      d. Patient is **uncomfortable** and **anxious** and has **tachycardia** and **hypertension.**
      e. **Holosystolic murmur** may be present, which indicates papillary muscle dysfunction secondary to ischemia.

   2. **MI is indicated by severe chest pain or pressure** that lasts **longer than 30 minutes.**
      a. **Nausea and vomiting** may be present.
      b. Patients are **diaphoretic** and **short of breath.**
      c. **Onset** is usually **at rest,** with **pain radiation** similar to that of angina.
      d. Patient often appears ill and has **tachycardia** and **hypertension** (hypotension may occur if infarction is substantial).
      e. **Signs and symptoms of CHF** may also be present.

C. Complications

   1. **MI may be silent and without consequence,** depending on the size of infarct.

   2. **Patients may develop CHF and pulmonary congestion.**

   3. **Hypotension** and **cardiogenic shock** may occur in significant infarction.

   4. **Acute onset of CHF** in conjunction with holosystolic murmur after MI usually indicates papillary muscle rupture with mitral valve insufficiency or ventricular septal rupture.

   5. **Life-threatening ventricular arrhythmias** are common in the first 24 hours after MI.

   6. **Inferior wall MIs** often produce sinus bradycardia and/or atrioventricular nodal block.

   7. **Bundle-branch blocks** are more likely with anterior MIs.

   8. **Left ventricular aneurysms** may lead to systemic emboli.

   9. **Pulmonary embolus (PE)** and **deep venous thrombosis (DVT)** may also occur.

D. Laboratory findings

   1. **ECG reveals evidence of MI** in 85% of patients.
      a. Initially, **ST segment elevation** occurs (current of injury or infarction) in leads associated with the infarcted area.
      b. **ST segments** then **begin to fall,** and **Q waves appear** along with inversion of T waves.

      c. **ST segment depression** occurs during angina, but often the ECG shows no significant changes.

    2. **Analysis of cardiac enzymes** reveals **elevated creatine kinase levels** (occur 6–12 hours after onset of infarction), followed by **elevated lactate dehydrogenase (LDH) levels** (occur > 24 hours after onset of infarction).

E. Treatment

    1. **Intravenous (IV) access, oxygen, and monitors** should be in place in any individual who has the appropriate history and signs and symptoms of MI.

    2. **Sublingual nitroglycerin** may relieve pain and reduce myocardial demand (this drug is **contraindicated in** patients who have **hypotension**).

    3. **Beta-blockers** are useful in **relieving tachycardia and hypertension,** thereby decreasing myocardial demand.

    4. **Morphine** may be necessary if nitroglycerin is ineffective.

    5. **Reduction of the infarcted tissue** can be achieved with early diagnosis (i.e., diagnosis within 6 hours of the onset of symptoms) through the use of **IV streptokinase or tissue plasminogen activator (t-PA).**

    6. **Prophylactic lidocaine** can be given for **arrhythmias.**

    7. Symptomatic **bradycardia** can be treated with **atropine** until a **transvenous pacemaker** is available.

    8. **Mitral regurgitation** can be treated with **arterial vasodilators** (e.g., nifedipine).

    9. **Initial heparinization and long-term anticoagulation (warfarin) therapy** is required in patients who develop **ventricular aneurysms, PE, and DVT.**

III. Valvular Heart Disease

A. The **most common valvular disorders** include aortic stenosis, aortic regurgitation, mitral stenosis, mitral regurgitation, and tricuspid regurgitation.

B. Aortic stenosis

    1. General characteristics

        a. Aortic stenosis is **most commonly caused by a congenital bicuspid aortic valve that** gradually **thickens and becomes stenotic** during adulthood.

        b. Aortic stenosis **may occur secondary to rheumatic fever,** but rarely without coexistent **mitral involvement.**

        c. The condition **affects more men than women** (ratio of 3:1).

        d. Aortic obstruction → **increased left ventricular pressure** → **left ventricular hypertrophy** (not dilatation, as in CHF).

    2. Clinical features

        a. **Angina** is a common symptom **due to increased myocardial oxygen demands.**

        b. **Syncope** during exercise occurs **due to the compensatory fall in peripheral resistance** combined with the inability of the heart to maintain adequate stroke volumes across the stenotic aortic valve.

        c. **Prolonged, severe pressure overload** occurs, which leads to CHF from myocardial dysfunction.

        d. **Delayed carotid upstroke, soft S_2** (due to decreased A_2 sound), **S_4 sound** (due to ventricular hypertrophy), and **systolic ejection murmur** are present.

        e. **Severe stenosis** puts patient at risk for sudden death.

3. Laboratory findings

a. ECG reveals evidence of **left ventricular hypertrophy** (nonspecific).

b. **Echocardiography** may reveal **calcified leaflets;** however, echocardiography **may not detect the degree of stenosis.**

c. **Cardiac catheterization** is the **definitive test.**

(1) Cardiac catheterization **reveals aortic orifice dimensions** through an evaluation of pressures across the aortic valve.

(2) However, improved **Doppler flow study** techniques have decreased the need for this procedure.

4. Treatment

a. **Cardiac catheterization** should be performed as soon as **syncope, angina, or left ventricular failure** appears in patients.

b. **Patients with good left ventricular function** have the lowest mortality during aortic valve replacement; **patients with poor ejection fractions** who survive surgery often respond well (i.e., poor left ventricular function is not a contraindication to surgery).

c. **Balloon valvuloplasty** can be effective **for** patients who are **poor surgical candidates (restenosis** is common).

C. Aortic regurgitation

1. General characteristics

a. Aortic regurgitation is **most commonly caused by rheumatic fever.**

b. This condition may also occur **secondary to infective endocarditis, hypertension, syphilis, or collagen vascular diseases.**

c. Aortic regurgitation → increased end-diastolic volume → ventricular dilatation → mitral regurgitation.

2. Clinical features

a. Patients have **signs and symptoms of left ventricular failure,** including orthopnea, dyspnea, and nocturia.

b. **Syncope** may occur due to decreased diastolic pressures secondary to regurgitation.

c. **Reduced diastolic pressures** also compromise coronary blood flow and occasionally present as angina.

d. **Additional signs** include laterally displaced point of maximal impulse, diastolic blowing murmur, and widened pulse pressure.

3. Laboratory findings

a. ECG is usually not helpful.

b. **Chest radiographic study** reveals **cardiac enlargement** with or without signs of pulmonary congestion; **dilated proximal aorta** may be seen.

c. **Echocardiography** reveals **enlarged left ventricle** with mitral valve vibration during diastole secondary to aortic regurgitation.

4. Treatment

a. **Surgical valve replacement** is indicated when **signs of decompensation** occur.

b. **Prosthetic valve replacement** requires **long-term anticoagulant therapy** and **antibiotic prophylaxis** for any operative procedure (including dental procedures).

c. **Arterial vasodilators, diuretics, and digitalis** (which increases cardiac contractility) may be used for symptomatic relief in patients who are **poor surgical candidates.**

D. Mitral stenosis

  1. General characteristics

   a. Mitral stenosis is **almost always due to rheumatic fever** and **usually occurs in women.**

   b. Mitral stenosis → increased left atrial pressure and enlargement → pulmonary venous congestion → pulmonary hypertension → right-sided failure.

  2. Clinical features

   a. When the **primary cause** is **childhood rheumatic fever, age of onset** of mitral stenosis is usually **between 24 and 45 years.**

   b. **Dyspnea and orthopnea** are common.

   c. **Right-sided failure** leads to ascites, edema, anorexia, and fatigue.

   d. **Hemoptysis** occurs secondary to increased pulmonary pressures and vessel rupture.

   e. Patients have an **irregular pulse** secondary to associated atrial fibrillation.

   f. **Systemic emboli** occur due to thrombi formed in the fibrillating atrium.

   g. **Additional signs** include increased S_1, increased P_2 (if pulmonary hypertension is present), opening snap following S_2, diastolic rumble, and inspiratory crackles (if pulmonary congestion is present).

  3. Laboratory findings

   a. **ECG** may reveal left atrial enlargement or atrial fibrillation.

   b. **Chest radiographic study** reveals atrial enlargement, pulmonary congestion, loss of retrosternal air space laterally (if right ventricular hypertrophy has occurred secondary to pulmonary hypertension).

   c. **Echocardiogram** often provides sufficient diagnostic imaging of the stenotic mitral valve; however, **cardiac catheterization** is still performed to assess other structures that may also be affected.

  4. Treatment

   a. Medical therapy includes **diuretic drugs** for patients who have pulmonary congestion and digitalis and **long-term anticoagulant therapy** (warfarin) for patients who have atrial fibrillation.

   b. To reduce operative mortality, **surgery** should be performed **before onset of pulmonary hypertension.**

    (1) Because **hypertension** does reverse upon correction of the defect, it is **not a contraindication to surgery.**

    (2) **Systemic embolization** despite anticoagulant therapy is an **indication for surgery.**

   c. **Mitral valvuloplasty** should be performed on patients who are **poor surgical candidates** (**restenosis** often occurs).

E. Mitral regurgitation

  1. General characteristics

   a. Mitral regurgitation is **most commonly caused by rheumatic fever** and is **more common in men.**

   b. The condition **can occur acutely with MI** if papillary muscle rupture occurs.

   c. Mitral regurgitation may also be seen **in mitral valve prolapse** and **hypertrophic cardiomyopathy,** or **secondary to cardiac dilatation.**

   d. Mitral regurgitation → increased left atrial pressure → increased pulmonary pressure → left ventricular dilatation (due to increased stroke volumes against the low resistance of the regurgitant mitral valve).

  2. Clinical features

   a. Signs include **dyspnea** and **orthopnea.**

b. **Pulmonary hypertension** and **right-sided failure** occur if regurgitation is severe and chronic.

c. **Atrial fibrillation** and **systemic emboli** may occur.

d. Additional signs include displaced point of maximal impulse, holosystolic apical murmur radiating to the axilla, and an S_3 sound (rapid filling of the left ventricle from the overloaded atrium).

3. Laboratory findings

a. **ECG** reveals evidence of left ventricular hypertrophy and enlargement.

b. **Chest radiographic study** reveals cardiac enlargement with or without pulmonary congestion.

c. **Echocardiography** shows regurgitant mitral valve and enlarged left-sided chambers.

4. Treatment

a. Because muscle dysfunction can occur, **mitral valve replacement** must be performed early.

b. **Medical therapy** includes:

(1) **Digitalis** for patients in atrial fibrillation or with cardiac muscle dysfunction

(2) **Diuretic drugs** for pulmonary congestion

(3) **Arterial vasodilators** to increase forward flow

(4) **Anticoagulant drugs** for patients with atrial fibrillation at risk of developing emboli

F. **Tricuspid regurgitation**

1. General characteristics

a. Tricuspid regurgitation is **usually secondary to right ventricular dilatation from pulmonary hypertension** and may therefore occur with **rheumatic fever.**

b. This condition should be **suspected in drug addicts who have infective endocarditis.**

c. Tricuspid regurgitation → increased right atrial pressure → venous hypertension.

2. Clinical features

a. **Signs and symptoms** are **similar to** those of **right-sided failure** (ascites and edema).

b. **Right upper quadrant pain** may occur **due to hepatic congestion** if condition develops acutely.

c. **Holosystolic murmur** is detected **along left sternal border.**

d. An additional sign is **elevated JVP during systole.**

e. Patients have **hepatojugular reflux** and a **pulsatile liver.**

3. Laboratory findings

a. **ECG** may reveal right ventricular and atrial enlargement.

b. **Chest radiographic study** reveals loss of retrosternal air space laterally, which indicates an enlarged right ventricle.

c. **Echocardiography** reveals enlarged right-sided chambers; **Doppler flow studies** can reveal the significance of the regurgitant valve.

4. Treatment

a. **Underlying disease** must be treated.

b. **Isolated tricuspid regurgitation** is usually well tolerated and **does not require surgery.**

IV. CARDIOMYOPATHIES AND PERICARDIAL DISEASE

A. General considerations

1. These **two clinical entities** are considered together because they often produce a **similar clinical picture.**

2. **Cardiomyopathies** include congestive cardiomyopathy, hypertrophic obstructive cardiomyopathy, and restrictive cardiomyopathy.

3. **Pericardial disease** can present as acute pericarditis, pericardial effusion, or constrictive pericarditis.

B. Congestive (dilated) cardiomyopathy

1. General characteristics

a. Congestive cardiomyopathy is a **loss of cardiac muscle function in the absence of pressure or volume overload and coronary artery disease;** that is, it is strictly caused by a malfunction of myocardium.

b. **Prolonged ethanol abuse** is the **most common cause.**

c. This condition may be **idiopathic or may be caused by infections or drugs** other than ethanol (e.g., doxorubicin).

d. Cardiac dilatation → left and right systolic dysfunction → congestive heart failure.

2. Clinical features

a. Signs and symptoms are **similar to those of congestive heart failure.**

b. **Murmur of mitral regurgitation** may be present secondary to dilatation.

3. Laboratory findings

a. ECG reveals nonspecific ST and T wave changes; left bundle-branch block is also common.

b. **Chest radiographic study** reveals cardiomegaly with pulmonary vascular congestion.

c. **Echocardiography** reveals dilated chambers with poor wall motion.

d. **Cardiac catheterization** is **not required for diagnosis.**

4. Treatment

a. If present, the **offending agent** (ethanol, other drugs) **should be withdrawn.**

b. **CHF** should be **treated with sodium restriction; diuretic drugs;** and **digitalis,** which improves contractility.

c. In selected patients, **cardiac transplantation** is effective.

C. Hypertrophic obstructive cardiomyopathy

1. General characteristics

a. This condition is also known as **idiopathic hypertrophic subaortic stenosis.**

b. Hypertrophy of interventricular septum → left ventricular outflow obstruction and impaired diastolic filling due to stiff left ventricle → pulmonary congestion.

c. Most cases are **autosomal dominant.**

2. Clinical features

a. **Dyspnea** is the **most common sign** and is **secondary to pulmonary congestion.**

b. **Angina** is often present.

c. Syncope after exercise occurs due to peripheral vasodilation, which decreases afterload → decreased left ventricular size → increased outflow obstruction.

d. **Carotid upstroke** has a spike and dome configuration.

e. **Systolic ejection murmur,** usually nonradiating, is detected along the left sternal border; **murmur increases** with maneuvers that decrease left ventricular size (e.g., **Valsalva's maneuver** or **standing**).

3. Laboratory findings
    a. **ECG** reveals hypertrophy of the left ventricle.
    b. **Echocardiography** is the best technique for visualizing the hypertrophic septum.
    c. **Cardiac catheterization** is used in patients who require quantification of the degree of obstruction before surgery or in patients whose septums are not well visualized by echocardiography.

4. Treatment
    a. **Medical therapy** is the standard approach.
        (1) **Beta-blockers** (e.g., propranolol) slow the heart rate and allow increased diastolic filling time, which diminishes the obstruction.
        (2) **Calcium channel blockers** (e.g., verapamil) improve ventricular compliance.
    b. **Surgical therapy** involves **myomectomy and/or mitral valve replacement** (the anterior leaflet of the mitral valve often produces obstruction); no evidence exists that surgery prolongs life in these patients.

D. Restrictive cardiomyopathy

1. General characteristics
    a. **Myocardium composition changes** → noncompliance → diastolic noncompliance with elevated filling pressures → pulmonary congestion.
    b. This condition is **less common than dilated or hypertrophic cardiomyopathies**.
    c. Restrictive cardiomyopathy is **often caused by an infiltrative process** (e.g., amyloidosis, sarcoidosis, hemochromatosis).

2. Clinical features
    a. **Signs and symptoms** are **similar to** those of **CHF.**
    b. **Kussmaul's sign** (an inspiratory increase in central venous pressure) may be present.

3. Laboratory findings
    a. **ECG** reveals low-voltage QRS complexes and nonspecific ST- and T-wave abnormalities.
    b. **Chest radiographic study** reveals pulmonary congestion without cardiomegaly.
    c. **Echocardiography** often reveals left ventricular thickening (left ventricular thickening in conjunction with low ECG voltages aids in diagnosis).
    d. **Cardiac catheterization** reveals unequal pressures in all four chambers **in contrast to constrictive pericarditis.**
    e. **Specific cause** is diagnosed through **tissue biopsy.**

4. Treatment
    a. The **underlying cause** must be treated, if possible.
    b. **Diuretic drugs** may alleviate symptoms of CHF.
    c. **Digitalis** may be used cautiously to increase contractility (these patients are sensitive to the drug's toxic effects).

E. Acute pericarditis

1. General characteristics
    a. Acute pericarditis is an **inflammation of the pericardium.**
    b. The disease may be **idiopathic or secondary to a viral infection** (e.g., coxsack-

ievirus B, hepatitis B, cytomegalovirus); **bacterial infection** (*Staphylococcus* sp, *Streptococcus* sp, tubercle bacillus); **post-MI complications; drugs** (e.g., procainamide); **malignancy** (usually pulmonary or breast metastases); or **collagen vascular disease** (e.g., systemic lupus erythematosus).

2. Clinical features
  a. Patients report **chest pain** that worsens with deep breathing, cough, and lying down and is relieved by sitting and leaning forward.
  b. **Pericardial friction rub** is heard in both systole and diastole; this finding **is diagnostic.**

3. Laboratory findings
  a. ECG reveals **ST segment elevation** in all precordial leads (Figure 4.2) without reciprocal ST segment depression (which occurs in MI).

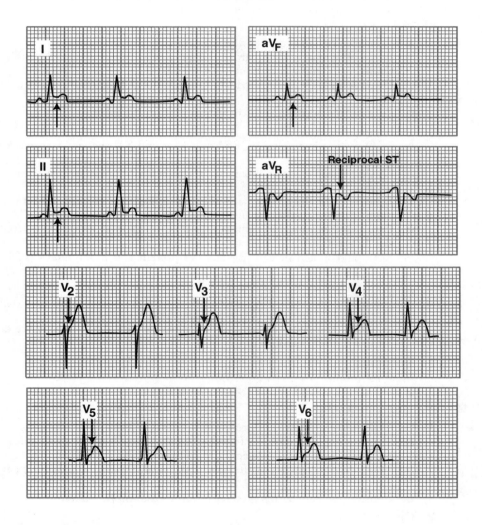

Figure 4-2. ECG of a patient who has acute pericarditis showing ST-segment elevation in all precordial leads (heavy arrow), but no reciprocal ST-segment depression.

   b. **Echocardiography** often reveals a **pericardial effusion,** which confirms the diagnosis.
4. Treatment
   a. The **underlying cause** must be treated.
   b. **Non-steroidal anti-inflammatory drugs (NSAIDs)** are usually effective in relieving pain and inflammation.
   c. Patients should be given **steroids** if they are unresponsive to NSAIDs.
   d. Results of **cardiac enzyme assays** are usually normal, but they may be helpful in ruling out MI.

F. Pericardial effusion
   1. General characteristics
      a. **Prolonged and/or severe inflammation** leads to an effusion.
      b. Rapid effusion leads to **cardiac tamponade,** but chronic accumulation is accommodated by the expanding pericardium.
   2. Clinical features
      a. **A small effusion** produces **no symptoms.**
      b. **Large effusions** lead to **cardiac tamponade** (hypotension, tachycardia, distended neck veins, indistinct heart sounds).
      c. **Heart sounds** are **diminished,** and it is difficult to locate the point of maximal impulse.
      d. **Friction rub secondary to coexistent pericarditis** is heard.
   3. Laboratory findings
      a. ECG reveals low-voltage QRS complexes and **ST changes associated with pericarditis.**
      b. **Cardiac shadow** has an enlarged "water-bottle" appearance **on chest radiograph.**
      c. **Echocardiography** may show an **anechoic space between the layers of pericardium;** this sign **is diagnostic** of pericardial effusion.
      d. **Pericardiocentesis,** the aspiration of fluid in the pericardial space, confirms the diagnosis.
         (1) Fluid should be sent for culture: **protein and LDH assays** (LDH and protein determine if fluid is a transudate or exudate); **cytology;** and **antinuclear antibody assay** (if collagen vascular disease is suspected).
         (2) **If tap is bloody, then let it clot.**
            (a) If it does not clot, then it is blood from the effusion.
            (b) If it does clot, then it is ventricular blood from a puncture during the procedure.
   4. Treatment
      a. If symptoms are severe, **pericardiocentesis** is indicated to remove fluid.
      b. Otherwise, therapy is the same as for acute pericarditis.

G. Constrictive pericarditis
   1. General characteristics
      a. Constrictive pericarditis is a **thickening and fibrosis of the pericardium that** occurs long after an acute episode of pericarditis.
      b. The condition can occur **after bacterial, viral, fungal, or neoplastic pericarditis.**
      c. Constrictive pericarditis **produces decreased diastolic filling.**
   2. Clinical features
      a. Patients report **dyspnea on exertion** and **orthopnea.**
      b. Edema, ascites, pulsatile liver, and elevated JVP are additional signs.

    c. The **volume of the carotid pulse** is decreased.

    d. **Heart sounds** are distant, and a **pericardial knock** is detected after S_2.

3. **Laboratory findings**

    a. **ECG** commonly reveals **low voltage in limb leads** and **atrial arrhythmias.**

    b. **Chest radiographic study** reveals **pericardial calcification.**

    c. **Echocardiography** is **often unreliable** diagnostically.

    d. **Cardiac catheterization** reveals **equal and elevated pressures in all four chambers** (unlike restrictive cardiomyopathy); **ventricular pressure tracings** reveal the **characteristic diastolic dip and systolic plateau** (square root sign).

4. **Treatment** is **pericardiectomy.**

V. DEEP VENOUS THROMBOSIS, PULMONARY EMBOLUS, AND AORTIC ANEURYSMS

A. Deep venous thrombosis (DVT)

1. **General characteristics**

    a. In DVT, a **blood clot forms** in the veins of the lower extremity or pelvis.

    b. DVT is **most often associated with prolonged immobilization** (e.g., extended postoperative period); **hypercoagulable states** (e.g., malignancies, estrogen use); **CHF;** and **varicose veins** (valvular insufficiency).

    c. DVT may not manifest until the patient presents with the **complication of PE.**

2. **Clinical features** include leg pain, swelling, warmth, and calf tenderness of the affected limb.

3. **Laboratory findings**

    a. **Doppler studies** are most effective in patients who have more proximal lesions; because these studies are noninvasive, they should be performed first.

    b. **Contrast venography** is the most effective method of delineating venous occlusion.

        (1) Contrast venography carries **risks,** because it is invasive and involves intravenous contrast material.

        (2) Contrast venography is **usually reserved for patients with symptoms highly suggestive of DVT** but whose **Doppler studies** are **inconclusive.**

4. **Treatment**

    a. **Intravenous heparin** is recommended for **patients with DVT proximal to the calf** (DVT below the knee generally does not require therapy) **until** the patient has undergone **anticoagulatation** [i.e., a partial thromboplastin time (PTT) 1.5 to 2.0 times the normal value, or an international normalized ratio (INR) between 2.0 and 3.0].

    b. The patient can then be maintained on **oral anticoagulation (warfarin) therapy** as prophylaxis for recurrent DVT (INR should be maintained between 2.0 and 2.5).

    c. When switching to oral therapy, the patient must be maintained on **intravenous heparin for 2 to 5 days after oral treatment** is initiated because of the lag that exists between the initiation of each therapy and attainment of its therapeutic effect.

    d. **Thrombolytic agents** (streptokinase, t-PA) have not been shown to significantly alter morbidity, mortality, or recurrence rates; therefore, these agents **are generally not used.**

B. Pulmonary embolus

1. General characteristics
   a. Pulmonary embolus results when a **thrombus** from a DVT **breaks off** and travels through the right-sided circulation and **becomes lodged** in the pulmonary artery.
   b. This condition produces **ventilation–perfusion mismatching** → **hypoxemia.**
   c. An **extensive embolus** may produce **pulmonary infarction** and **right ventricular overload.**

2. Clinical features
   a. **Dyspnea** is the most common sign.
   b. Additional signs and symptoms include pleuritic chest pain, tachypnea, and hemoptysis.
   c. **Syncope** may occur if PE is extensive and compromises cardiac output.
   d. Patients are **tachycardic** and have a **low-grade fever** (<38.0°C).
   e. **Splinting, wheezing,** and a **pleural effusion** may be detected.
   f. In **massive PE, right-sided heart failure** and a **loud P$_2$** are evident.
   g. **Evidence of a DVT** may be present, which should alert the physician to the **diagnosis** of PE.

3. Laboratory findings
   a. **ECG** often reveals only **sinus tachycardia,** but may also show **poor R wave progression** in anterior leads.
   b. **Chest radiographic study** may reveal **decreased vascular markings** in the area of the obstruction; a **wedge-shaped pleural-based density** is a classic sign if **pulmonary infarction** has occurred and may be associated with a **pleural effusion** (Figure 4-3).
   c. Results of **arterial blood gas studies** may indicate hypoxia, hypocarbia (due to hyperventilation), and respiratory alkalosis; however, these **changes** are **not specific to PE** and may not necessarily be present.
   d. **Normal ventilation–perfusion scan results rule out** the **diagnosis** of PE.
      (1) However, the results are often of intermediate probability (i.e., PE diagnosis cannot be confirmed or ruled out).
      (2) Ventilation–perfusion scan should be performed if the situation is not emergent, because this procedure carries less risk than pulmonary angiography.
   e. **Pulmonary angiography** (arteriography) is the **gold standard** for diagnosis of PE; this procedure requires a pulmonary artery catheter and contrast material and therefore carries some risk.
   f. **Digital subtraction angiography** is a new test that requires only a small amount of contrast material injected intravenously (i.e., this test obviates pulmonary vessel catheterization).

4. Treatment
   a. Patients should receive **oxygen by mask.**
   b. **IV heparin** should be given for **7 to 10 days** to maintain the PTT between 1.5 and 2.0 times the normal value; in patients who have clinical symptoms that strongly suggest the diagnosis, heparin should be started before diagnostic confirmation.
   c. **Oral anticoagulation therapy** can be started before heparin is discontinued to maintain PT at 1.3 to 1.5 times baseline (INR, 2.0 to 3.0).
   d. Patients who have **massive embolus may benefit from thrombolytic agents** (streptokinase or t-PA).
   e. If **anticoagulation is contraindicated** (e.g., recent or ongoing hemorrhage) **or**

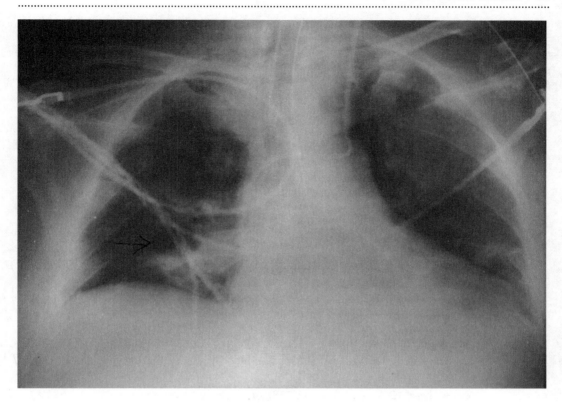

Figure 4-3. The uncommonly seen appearance of pulmonary embolism on radiographic chest film. Note the opacity in the right lower lobe. This nonspecific finding could represent an infectious infiltrate; however, this patient's ventilation-perfusion scan reveals that the patient has had a pulmonary embolism. (Reprinted with permission from Freundlich IM, Bragg DG: *A Radiologic Approach to Diseases of the Chest*, 2nd ed. Baltimore, Williams & Wilkins, p 410.)

if the patient shows evidence of recurrent PE despite heparin therapy in the initial 24 hours, a **venacaval interruption** (with a Greenfield filter) may be performed.

C. Aortic aneurysms

    1. General characteristics

        a. Aortic aneurysms may occur in the ascending aorta, aortic arch, descending aorta, or abdominal aorta.

        b. The **most common cause** of aortic aneurysm is **atherosclerotic disease** leading to abdominal aortic aneurysm; this type is **usually seen in older men.**

    2. Clinical features

        a. The condition is **usually asymptomatic until rupture occurs,** or the aneurysm may be perceived as an **abdominal fullness or pulsation.**

        b. **Back and epigastric pain** may be present, which becomes **severe before rupture.**

        c. A **pulsatile abdominal mass** may be palpated.

        d. Evidence of **peripheral emboli** may be present.

  e. Symptoms of associated **peripheral vascular disease** (e.g., intermittent claudication) are **common.**

  f. Aneurysm may **rupture** into the gastrointestinal (GI) tract in the form of acute massive GI hemorrhage.

   (1) Ruptures into the retroperitoneal space produce **flank or groin hematomas.**

   (2) Ruptures into the abdominal cavity produce **abdominal distention.**

3. Laboratory findings

 a. **Abdominal ultrasound** is effective in detecting and measuring the diameter of aortic aneurysms.

 b. **Angiography** is necessary to define surgical anatomy.

4. Treatment

 a. Surgery is recommended **for aneurysms > 6 cm** in size and for **patients whose aneurysms have ruptured.**

 b. **Poor surgical candidates with aneurysms between 4 and 6 cm can be followed up closely,** because these aneurysms rupture less frequently than larger aneurysms; however, these patients require **surgery if the aneurysm expands or signs of impending rupture** occur.

VI. SYSTEMIC HYPERTENSON

A. **General characteristics**

1. Systemic hypertension is defined as **blood pressure** that is consistently **> 140/90 mm Hg.**

2. At least **15% of whites and 25% of blacks** are hypertensive.

3. Hypertension may be **essential (primary)** or **secondary.**

4. **Diagnosis** is made when the patient has at least two consistently elevated blood pressure readings on separate occasions, with the patient at rest for at least 15 minutes before measurement.

B. **Essential (primary) hypertension**

1. General characteristics

 a. Essential hypertension is defined as hypertension that occurs **without any identifiable cause.**

 b. **Ninety to ninety-five percent** of hypertensive patients fall into this category.

 c. Essential hypertension is **usually detected during middle age.**

 d. If the condition is **not treated,** the **mortality rate increases dramatically** due to stroke, coronary artery disease, and/or congestive heart failure.

 e. **Retinal hemorrhages** indicate more severe disease.

 f. **Malignant hypertension** is a **rapidly progressive form of essential hypertension** with diastolic readings > 120 mm Hg and widespread end-organ dysfunction.

2. Clinical features

 a. Patients are **often asymptomatic until** they are seen with **complications** as described previously.

 b. Patients who have malignant hypertension may report **blurred vision, headache, and dyspnea.**

  (1) **Papilledema, fundal hemorrhages,** and **infarctions** (cotton wool spots) are additional signs.

(2) Encephalopathy may develop.

(3) Renal damage with microangiopathic hemolytic anemia is common.

3. Laboratory findings

a. Patients who have hypertension should have **baseline studies** to give an **indication of end-organ function.**

b. Studies should include **ECG; complete blood count; urinalysis;** and **serum studies,** including electrolytes, creatinine, urea, glucose (to check for possible coexisting diabetes), triglycerides, cholesterol, and uric acid.

4. Treatment

a. Treatment should be **aimed at reducing diastolic pressures to < 90 mm Hg.**

b. **Limiting dietary sodium to < 2 g/day** may be sufficient and should constitute the **first line of therapy** unless more severe disease is present.

c. **Diuretic drugs (thiazides)** decrease plasma volume and vascular resistance; diuretics may cause hypokalemia and hyperuricemia, which may necessitate the use of **potassium supplements.**

d. **Beta-blockers** (e.g., propranolol) reduce cardiac output and decrease renin-angiotensin–mediated sodium and water reabsorption; **side effects** include worsening CHF, occasional vascular incompetence, fatigue, depression, and nightmares.

e. **Vasodilators (hydralazine, minoxidil)** are **effective** when used **with β-blockers;** β-blockers **inhibit the reflex tachycardia** that can occur **with vasodilators.**

f. **Methyldopa and clonidine** (centrally acting adrenergic agonists) may be effective in cases where β-blockers are relatively **contraindicated.**

g. **Prazosin and phenoxybenzamine (α-blockers)** are used less commonly.

h. **Angiotensin converting enzyme (ACE) inhibitors** such as captopril are effective in **reducing hypertension** and may be **cardioprotective; side effects** include leukopenia, rashes, cough, and proteinuria.

i. **Therapeutic approach** consists of first instituting **dietary measures.** If these measures fail, institute **diuretic drug therapy;** then, add a β-blocker if required, followed by a vasodilator, and then followed by captopril or an α-blocker.

C. Secondary hypertension

1. General characteristics

a. Secondary hypertension is seen in **5% to 10% of patients who have hypertension.**

b. Secondary hypertension should be **suspected if hypertension appears in a young person or in a person who does not respond to treatments for primary hypertension.**

c. **Important treatable causes** include **renovascular hypertension and pheochromocytoma.**

d. Other causes include **renal parenchymal disease** (acute or chronic), **oral contraceptive use** (hypertension occurs in 5% of users and is reversible upon discontinuation of the preparation), **primary aldosteronism, Cushing's syndrome,** and **hyperparathyroidism.**

2. Renovascular hypertension

a. General characteristics

(1) Obstruction of renal blood flow $\rightarrow$ perceived as volume depletion by kidney $\rightarrow$ stimulation of the renin-angiotensin-aldosterone system $\rightarrow$ increased sodium and water reabsorption $\rightarrow$ hypertension.

(2) This disease is **often caused by atherosclerotic disease in the elderly or fibromuscular disease of the renal artery in young women.**

   b. A clinical feature is **abdominal bruit** over the renal artery.

   c. Laboratory findings

      (1) **Renal arteriogram** reveals a **stenotic lesion, which is diagnostic.**

      (2) **Renal vein renin tests** reveal **increased renin** in samples drawn from renal vein **ipsilateral to the stenosis** compared with samples drawn from the contralateral side (if the contralateral side is unaffected).

      (3) **Elevated serum urea level** is indicative of **decreased renal perfusion.**

   d. Treatment

      (1) Medical therapy consisting of **ACE inhibitors and other antihypertensives** is used **in poor surgical candidates.**

      (2) **Transluminal angioplasty or surgical revascularization** is often curative in operable candidates.

3. **Pheochromocytoma** is a tumor of the adrenal gland that produces norepinephrine.

   a. Clinical features

      (1) Signs and symptoms include **paroxysmal sweating, flushing, and palpitations.**

      (2) **Orthostatic hypotension with intermittent hypertension** is present.

   b. Laboratory findings

      (1) **Urinalysis** reveals increased catecholamine, metanephrine, and vanillylmandelic acid levels.

      (2) **Computed tomographic scan of the abdomen** often reveals the tumor.

   c. Treatment is **surgical removal of the tumor** following preoperative blood pressure control with α-blockers.

5

Pulmonary Diseases

I. OBSTRUCTIVE LUNG DISEASE

A. These diseases are **characterized by decreased expiratory flow rates** and include asthma, chronic obstructive pulmonary disease, bronchiectasis, and cystic fibrosis.

B. Asthma

1. General characteristics

a. Asthma is characterized by **hyperirritable airways** → **reversible airway obstruction.**

b. Asthma occurs in **5% to 10% of the population.**

c. The **intrinsic form** occurs in adults and is not associated with specific inhaled triggers.

d. The **extrinsic (allergic) form** occurs more commonly in children and is triggered by specific inhaled substances.

2. Clinical features

a. Patients experience **episodic bouts of coughing, dyspnea, expiratory wheezing,** and **chest tightness.**

b. Symptoms worsen with exercise, inhaling cold air or irritating gases, upper respiratory tract infections, and emotional stress.

c. **Tachycardia, tachypnea** with prolonged expiration, and **overinflation of chest** occur during episodes.

d. **Status asthmaticus** is a prolonged, **severe** asthmatic **attack that does not respond to initial bronchodilator therapy.**

(1) Status asthmaticus leads to **fatigue, cyanosis, tachycardia,** and **pulsus paradoxus** (decrease in systolic blood pressure >15 mm Hg with inspiration).

(2) These patients are **at risk for respiratory failure and death.**

3. Laboratory findings

a. **Pulmonary function tests** reveal **decreased** forced expiratory volume in 1 second (**FEV$_1$**), **hyperinflation** that improves with inhalation by a bronchodilating drug, and **increased total lung capacity (TLC) and residual lung volume** (RV).

b. **Methacoline** and **cold-air challenge tests** produce bronchoconstriction in patients who have asthma at doses lower than those that produce bronchoconstriction in persons whose airways are functioning normally.

c. **Sputum culture** should be performed to **rule out infectious etiology** (especially *Aspergillus fumigatus*); sputum culture of asthma patients **may contain increased eosinophils.**

    d. **Serum analysis** reveals **leukocytosis** with increased eosinophils.

    e. **Chest radiographic findings** reveal **hyperinflation.**

    f. **Arterial blood gas (ABG) analysis** usually indicates a **decreased PaCO$_2$ level** (<36 mm Hg) due to hyperventilation.

        (1) Hypoxia still occurs despite hyperventilation due to ventilation–perfusion mismatch.

        (2) Elevated PaCO$_2$ level indicates severe obstruction; these patients will develop a mixed respiratory and metabolic acidosis due to hypercapnia and lactic acidosis caused by decreased oxygen delivery.

4. Treatment

    a. Patients should be instructed to **avoid trigger agents.**

    b. **Cromolyn sodium** (mast cell stabilizer) can prevent an attack if administered before exposure to the trigger.

        (1) This drug is **ineffective if the attack has begun.**

        (2) This drug is **most effective in young patients** who have the **extrinsic form** of asthma.

    c. **Nebulized sympathomimetics** (e.g., metaproterenol, albuterol) relax bronchial smooth muscle and decrease airway obstruction; the **"albuterol puffer"** is usually the first line of therapy.

    d. **Corticosteroids** should be used for acute, severe exacerbations.

    e. **Aminophylline** can be given intravenously for acute, severe episodes.

C. Chronic obstructive pulmonary disease (COPD)

1. General characteristics

    a. COPD is a **progressive airway obstruction.**

    b. COPD affects **middle-aged and older individuals.**

    c. **Emphysema** (abnormal enlargement of air spaces with destruction of alveolar walls) and **chronic bronchitis** (productive cough for at least 3 months during each of 2 consecutive years) are **hallmarks** of the disease.

    d. COPD is most commonly associated with a **significant smoking history.**

2. Clinical features

    a. COPD has an **insidious onset.**

    b. **Chronic cough** eventually progresses to **dyspnea** on exertion.

    c. Unlike asthma, the **degree of airway obstruction** in COPD does not fluctuate as widely.

    d. **Exacerbations** can occur with respiratory tract infections, trauma, or surgery.

    e. **Signs of hyperinflation, use of accessory respiratory muscles,** and **diffuse wheezing** are present.

    f. Two clinically distinct **types of COPD patients** exist.

        (1) **"Pink puffers"** often present in later years (>60 years of age) with progressive dyspnea and weight loss, but little cough or sputum; these patients have **mild hypoxia** and **hypocapnia with overinflation** and show **little improvement with bronchodilator therapy.**

        (2) **"Blue bloaters"** present at an **earlier age** with **chronic cough** and **expectoration, weight gain,** and **episodic dyspnea;** these patients have **severe hypoxia** that leads to **polycythemia,** and they **respond well to bronchodilator therapy.**

        (3) **Most patients** are seen to have some **combination** of both entities.

    g. Chronic hypoxia → **pulmonary arterial constriction and pulmonary hypertension** → **right-sided failure** (cor pulmonale).

    h. Patients may develop **spontaneous pneumothorax secondary to emphysematous bullous disease,** especially secondary to mechanical ventilation.

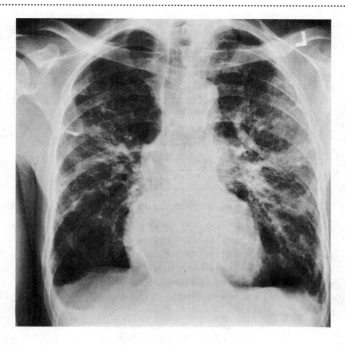

Figure 5-1. Chest film of a patient with long-standing chronic obstructive pulmonary disease. Note the hyperinflated lungs and flattened diaphragm. This patient also has a right lower pneumothorax that can occur spontaneously in such patients. (Reprinted with permission from Freundlich IM, Bragg DG: *A Radiologic Approach to Diseases of the Chest*, 2nd ed. Baltimore, Williams & Wilkins, p 357.)

3. Laboratory findings
  a. **Spirometry** is a useful **screening tool** that reveals decreased FEV_1 to forced vital capacity (FVC) ratios.
  b. **Pulmonary function tests** reveal **decreased vital capacity and expiratory flow rates** with **increased RV and TLC; improvement with bronchodilators** may occur, but improvement is often no more than 15% to 20% (**less than that seen with asthma**).
  c. **ABG analysis** indicates **hypoxia with hypocapnia** early in the disease and **hypercapnia** as the disease becomes more severe.
  d. **Chest radiographic study** reveals overinflation, bronchial thickening, and emphysematous bullae (Figure 5-1).

4. Treatment
  a. **Prevention** can be achieved with **smoking cessation.**
  b. **Beta-adrenergic agonists** (see asthma, I B 3 c) often provide **short-term relief.**
  c. **Corticosteroids** are usually reserved for patients who have **more severe disease** and/or exacerbations.
  d. **Annual vaccinations** for **pneumococcal and influenza infection** are necessary to **prevent respiratory tract infections that can be fatal** in such compromised patients.
  e. **Resection of emphysematous bullae** can be performed in **low-risk surgical candidates.**
  f. **Lung transplantation** is a new mode of therapy.

D. Bronchiectasis

   1. General characteristics
      a. Bronchiectasis is an **abnormal dilatation of the bronchi.**
      b. This disease is usually **secondary to severe necrotizing lung infection** (usually gram-negative organisms) associated with aspiration, or **anatomic disruption from a lung tumor** leading to recurrent pulmonary infections.

   2. Clinical features
      a. Patients have a **chronic cough** with large amounts of **foul-smelling, blood-tinged sputum.**
      b. **Progressive dyspnea** occurs.
      c. **Persistent crackles** are heard, and **pleuritic pain** is present over the affected lung field(s).
      d. **Clubbing** and **cor pulmonale** occur in long-standing disease.

   3. Laboratory findings
      a. **Pulmonary function tests** may reveal a restrictive pattern (increased FEV_1 with decreased lung volumes) or a mixture of restrictive and obstructive patterns.
      b. **Chest radiographic study** reveals peribronchial thickening with collapsed areas of lung in the regions of bronchiectasis (Figure 5-2).
      c. **Bronchoscopy** is a new diagnostic tool that provides direct visualization of the affected regions.
      d. Although **bronchography** is also a useful diagnostic tool, this test requires contrast medium and should be performed only in a patient who is unstable and has no infections; this test **is rarely indicated.**
      e. **Computed tomographic (CT) scan** is often sufficient to visualize the lesions.

   4. Treatment
      a. Patients should receive appropriate **antibiotic therapy** on a regular basis (ampicillin, tetracycline, erythromycin).
      b. **Associated abscesses** should be **drained.**
      c. Patients should receive **annual pneumococcal and influenza vaccines.**
      d. **Surgery** is usually of **little benefit.**

E. Cystic fibrosis (CF)

   1. General characteristics
      a. CF is an **autosomal recessive disease.**
      b. In CF, **exocrine gland dysfunction** → obstruction of **secretory glands** of the lung, pancreas, and gastrointestinal tract.
      c. CF is the **most common cause of obstructive airway disease in persons under** 30 years of age.

   2. Clinical features
      a. The disease usually manifests itself in childhood as **steatorrhea** or **bowel obstruction.**
      b. CF is seen as **meconium ileus in the neonate.**
      c. **Additional signs** include sinusitis, nasal polyps, and clubbing.
      d. Later, **recurrent lung infections** with *Staphylococcus aureus* and *Pseudomonas aeruginosa* are the major problem.
      e. CF causes **sterility in men.**
      f. **Cor pulmonale** (manifesting as right-sided heart failure) develops **secondary to pulmonary hypertension,** which results from areas of **hypoventilation.**

   3. Laboratory findings
      a. **Sweat test** reveals elevated sweat chloride levels (>60 mEq/L).

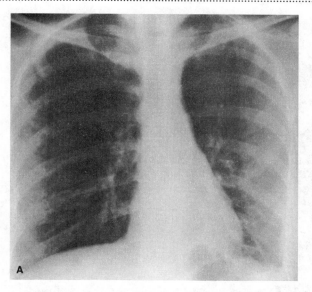

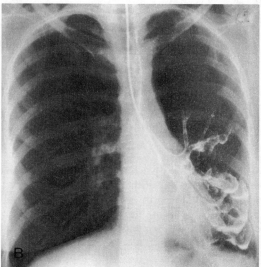

Figure 5-2.   **A,** Plain film of a patient with bronchiectasis. Some left lower lobe volume loss with hyperlucent areas is evident. **B,** Bronchogram delineating cystic bronchiectasis in the same patient. (Reprinted with permission from Freundlich IM, Bragg DG: A *Radiologic Approach to Diseases of the Chest,* 2nd ed. Baltimore, Williams & Wilkins, p 716.)

      b. **Pulmonary function tests** reveal an obstructive pattern with decreased expiratory flow rates and increased RV.

      c. **Chest radiographic study** reveals hyperinflation, cyst formation, bronchiectasis, and atelectasis (Figure 5-3).

   4. Treatment

      a. **Salt depletion** may occur; patients **may require supplements.**

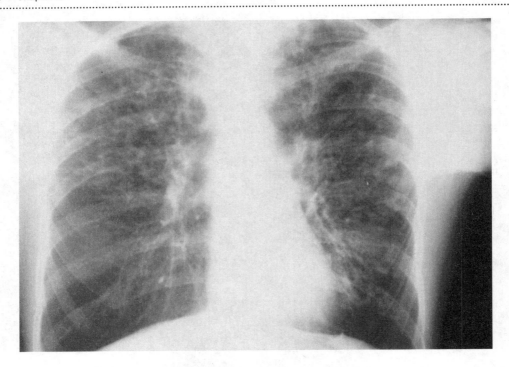

Figure 5-3. Chest radiographic study of a patient who has cystic fibrosis. The upper lung zones show evidence of fibrosis and bronchiectasis with peribronchial cuffing. The lower lung segments are commonly involved late in the disease. (Reprinted with permission from Freundlich IM, Bragg DG: *A Radiologic Approach to Diseases of the Chest,* 2nd ed. Baltimore, Williams & Wilkins, p 19.)

  b. Patients should receive **pancreatic enzyme replacement.**
  c. Patients need **chest physiotherapy** to assist with clearing of secretions.
  d. **Antibiotics** (cephalosporin or penicillin with an aminoglycoside) and **oxygen** are given for acute, severe infections.
  e. **Bronchodilators** are of some benefit when bronchospasm is prominent.
  f. **Lobectomy** is occasionally required for localized infection or tissue destruction.

II. DIFFUSE INTERSTITIAL LUNG DISEASE

A. General characteristics

 1. These disorders are characterized by an **infiltration of the lung parenchyma that** eventually leads to **pulmonary fibrosis.**

 2. The **most common entities** include idiopathic pulmonary fibrosis, pneumoconiosis, hypersensitivity pneumonitis, and sarcoidosis.

B. Idiopathic pulmonary fibrosis

 1. General characteristics
  a. Idiopathic pulmonary fibrosis **usually occurs in middle-aged persons.**

    b. No predisposing factor has been found.

    c. The disease may **progress rapidly or slowly.**

  2. Clinical features

    a. Constitutional signs and symptoms of **fatigue, fever,** and **weight loss** are common.

    b. Patients experience **dyspnea upon exertion.**

    c. A **nonproductive cough** is present.

    d. **Additional signs** include tachypnea, inspiratory crackles, small tidal volumes, and digital clubbing.

    e. Evidence of **right-sided heart failure** and **cyanosis** occur **in severe disease.**

  3. Laboratory findings

    a. **Pulmonary function tests** reveal small lung volumes and increased expiratory flow rates (increased FEV_1 to FVC ratio); these results are **not specific to the cause** of the pulmonary fibrosis and only **indicate the restrictive component of the lung disease.**

    b. **Chest radiographic study** reveals a diffuse reticulonodular pattern.

    c. **Open-lung biopsy** is required for **definitive diagnosis.**

  4. Treatment

    a. **Corticosteroids** are the mainstay of therapy.

    b. **Azathioprine or cyclophosphamide** is used in **steroid-resistant disease.**

C. Pneumoconiosis

  1. General characteristics

    a. **Pneumoconiosis** results from inhalation of organic dust (e.g., asbestos, silica, metals).

    b. **Asbestos exposure** is **associated with increased incidence of bronchogenic carcinoma and mesotheliomas** (especially if the patient smokes).

    c. Often, the disease has a **prolonged latency period** after exposure.

    d. **Silicosis** is associated with superinfection by **Mycobacterium tuberculosis.**

  2. Clinical features

    a. Patients usually have a **progressive fibrosis of the lung** that leads to **increasing dyspnea and cough.**

    b. **Signs and symptoms similar** to those of **idiopathic pulmonary fibrosis** occur.

  3. Laboratory findings

    a. **Pulmonary function tests** reveal a restrictive pattern, as in idiopathic pulmonary fibrosis.

    b. **Chest radiographic study** depends on the offending agent.

      (1) **Diffuse reticulonodular pattern** is seen in **coal dust exposure.**

      (2) **Perihilar egg-shell calcifications** are seen in **silicosis.**

      (3) **Calcified plaques** and **pleural thickening** are seen in **asbestos exposure** with or without evidence of **bronchogenic carcinoma or mesothelioma.**

    c. **Tissue biopsy** often reveals the offending agent.

  4. Treatment

    a. Patients should **avoid exposure** to the **offending agent.**

    b. Patients should **stop smoking.**

    c. **Coexisting tuberculosis** should be **treated** (e.g., with isoniazid).

    d. **Oxygen** should be given if disease impairs oxygenation and/or progresses to cor pulmonale.

D. Hypersensitivity pneumonitis

  1. General characteristics

    a. Hypersensitivity pneumonitis occurs in persons who have an **abnormal sensitivity to an organic agent.**

    b. Examples include **farmer's lung** (caused by exposure to Actinomyces in moldy hay) and **pigeon-breeder's lung** (caused by exposure to animal protein in bird droppings).

  2. Clinical features

    a. Patients experience onset of **cough, dyspnea, fever,** and **malaise** several hours after exposure; **symptoms slowly resolve** but **recur upon re-exposure.**

    b. **Diffuse crackles** can be heard, but wheezing usually is not present (unlike asthma).

    c. **Duration of symptoms** may increase with repeated exposure, eventually **leading to pulmonary fibrosis.**

  3. Laboratory findings

    a. **Chest radiographic study** reveals reticulonodular infiltrates, with sparing of the apices.

    b. **Hematology studies** reveal leukocytosis after exposure (eosinophilia is not seen).

    c. **Serum precipitins** to the offending agent are often present (their presence is not specific to the disease but does indicate exposure to the offending agent).

    d. **Pulmonary function tests** may reveal a **restrictive pattern.**

    e. **Transbronchial biopsy** or **open-lung biopsy tissue** may be required for **definitive diagnosis.**

  4. Treatment

    a. Patient should **avoid exposure** to the offending agent.

    b. **Corticosteroids** may be required **in the acute phase** and may be of some benefit **in patients who progress to chronic, severe fibrosis.**

E. Sarcoidosis

  1. General characteristics

    a. Sarcoidosis is a condition in which **noncaseating granulomas** occur throughout the body **in association with a T-cell abnormality.**

    b. The disease is **most common in blacks in the third to fourth decade** of life.

  2. Clinical features

    a. **Fifty percent** of patients present with **pulmonary disease** consisting of progressive, nonproductive cough and shortness of breath, and/or laryngeal or endobronchial obstruction.

    b. **Other patients** present with **constitutional symptoms** (fever, malaise).

    c. **Pleurisy** and **hemoptysis** are **uncommon.**

    d. **Other clinical features** include:

      (1) **Uveitis** that may progress to blindness

      (2) Various **infiltrative lesions** and **erythema nodosum**

      (3) **Polyarthritis** and **cystic destruction of bone**

      (4) **Cranial neuropathies** (e.g., Bell's palsy) and **peripheral neuropathies**

      (5) **Arrhythmias** and **conduction disturbances**

      (6) Increased formation of **1,25-dihydroxyvitamin D,** which leads to hypercalcemia, hypercalciuria, and renal stones

  3. Laboratory findings

    a. **Pulmonary function tests** reveal a tendency toward a restrictive pattern and impaired diffusing capacity.

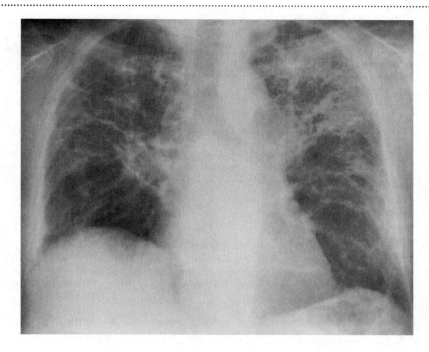

Figure 5-4.   Marked hilar and paratracheal lymphadenopathy in a patient who has sarcoidosis. Also note the bilateral reticulonodular pattern. (Reprinted with permission from Freundlich IM, Bragg DG: *A Radiologic Approach to Diseases of the Chest*, 2nd ed. Baltimore, Williams & Wilkins, p 182.)

    b. Chest radiographic study reveals hilar lymphadenopathy, diffuse nodular infiltrates, fibrosis, and honeycombing (Figure 5-4).

    c. Transbronchial biopsy or **tissue biopsy** confirms the diagnosis by revealing typical granulomas.

    d. Sputum cultures should be obtained before biopsy to rule out infectious etiology (e.g., tuberculosis).

4. Treatment

    a. Corticosteroids are first-line therapy if symptoms cause significant morbidity.

    b. Patients must be followed up with **regular pulmonary function tests** and **chest radiographic studies** in order to determine the need for continuation of treatment.

    c. Most patients have a **good prognosis,** with disease regression within 2 to 3 years.

III. ADULT RESPIRATORY DISTRESS SYNDROME (ARDS)

A. General characteristics

    1. ARDS is an **acute respiratory failure** characterized by hypoxemia, bilateral pulmonary infiltrates, and decreased lung compliance without preceding lung disease.

    2. ARDS may be seen in **association** with disseminated intravascular coagulopathy, bacterial septicemia, trauma, blood transfusions, pancreatitis, and smoke inhalation.

B. Clinical features

1. **Accumulation of pulmonary fluid** leads to dyspnea and hyperventilation.

2. **Without treatment,** patients progress to **respiratory failure within 24 hours.**

C. Laboratory findings

1. **Chest radiographic study** reveals a fine, diffuse, reticular infiltrate.

2. **ABG analysis** reveals hypoxia and hypocarbia initially and **hypercarbia** as respiratory failure ensues.

3. **No specific diagnostic test** exists; the diagnosis is based on the clinical presentation and is achieved after infectious etiology is ruled out.

D. Treatment

1. The **underlying cause** must be **treated.**

2. Patients should receive **adequate oxygen** (tracheal intubation if necessary) with high FIO_2 (inspired oxygen) initially.
   a. **High-concentration oxygen** must be reduced as soon as possible due to the toxicities associated with this oxygen therapy.
   b. $FIO_2 > 0.60$ can be tolerated for up to approximately 24 hours.

3. **Positive pressure ventilation** is often required due to reduced lung compliance.

4. **Corticosteroids** are **not beneficial** in the treatment of ARDS and are contraindicated if the condition is secondary to bacterial sepsis.

5. **Empiric antibiotic therapy** should be started if no other etiology for the condition is found.

IV. DISORDERS OF THE PLEURAL SPACE, MEDIASTINUM, AND CHEST WALL

A. Pleural diseases

1. Pleural effusions
   a. General characteristics
      (1) Pleural effusions are either **transudative or exudative.**
      (2) Determining whether an effusion is a transudate or an exudate allows the clinician to narrow the diagnostic possibilities (Tables 5-1 and 5-2).
   b. Clinical features
      (1) **Dyspnea** is a common sign.
      (2) Patients report **chest discomfort** that is often pleuritic.
      (3) **Vocal fremitus** and **breath sounds** are decreased over the effusion.
      (4) **Percussion** is dull over the effusion.

Table 5-1
Exudative Versus Transudative Fluid

	Exudate	Transudate
Protein content	<3 g/dl	>3 g/dl
Pleural: serum protein ratio	>0.5	<0.5
LDH content	>200 U/L	<200 U/L
Pleural: serum LDH level	>0.6	<0.6

Table 5-2
Differential Diagnosis of Pleural Effusions

Transudates	Exudates

CHF
Hypoalbuminemia (e.g.,
  nephrotic syndrome,
  starvation, cirrhosis)
	Bacterial infection (e.g., Actinomyces, Tuberculosis, Mycoplasma)
	Malignancy (e.g., bronchogenic carcinoma, mesothelioma, metastases)
	Pulmonary embolus
	Rheumatoid arthritis
	SLE
	Drug-induced (e.g., quinidine)
	Abdominal process (e.g., pancreatitis, subphrenic abscess)
	Trauma (e.g., hemothorax, chylothorax, ruptured esophagus)

(5) **Other signs and symptoms** associated with the specific cause must be sought (e.g., fever and productive cough suggest an infectious etiology).

c. Laboratory findings

(1) If more tha 250 ml of fluid are present, the fluid may appear on **chest radiographic study** as blunting of the costophrenic angle or as a concave meniscus.

(2) A **subpulmonic effusion** may be mistaken for an **elevated hemidiaphragm** (easily distinguished by a lateral decubitus film).

(3) **CT scan** may be necessary if the patient has **coexisting parenchymal disease;** coexisting disease makes it difficult to distinguish the presence of an effusion.

(4) **Aspirate from thoracocentesis** should be sent **for protein and lactate dehydrogenase analysis** (these analyses distinguish transudate from exudate—see Table 5-1), followed by further analyses, such as **cytology** (e.g., for suspected malignancy) and **culture and sensitivity** (e.g., for suspected infection).

(5) **Special investigations** can suggest **specific diagnoses:**

(a) Presence of **leukoerythrogenic cells** suggests systemic lupus erthyematosus **(SLE).**

(b) Presence of **rheumatoid factor** suggests **rheumatoid arthritis.**

(c) **Glucose < 20 mg/dl** is consistent with **rheumatoid arthritis.**

(d) **Amylase levels** more than twice the normal value suggest **esophageal perforation** or **pancreatitis.**

(e) **Hematocrit > 20%** suggests **hemothorax** (suspect malignancy, trauma, or pulmonary embolus).

(f) **High lymphocyte count** (>50% of white blood cells) suggests **tuberculosis** or **malignancy.**

(g) **Pleural fluid pH measurements** are usually of **little clinical value.**

d. Treatment

(1) The **underlying cause** must be **treated.**

(2) Symptomatic improvement can be achieved with **fluid aspiration,** but relief is only temporary.

(3) **Empyemas** must be **drained.**

(4) **Repeated thoracocentesis should be avoided,** because this procedure results in significant protein depletion.

(5) **Chemical pleurodesis** (intrapleural tetracycline) can benefit patients who have **malignant effusions.**

2. Pneumothorax

a. **General characteristics**

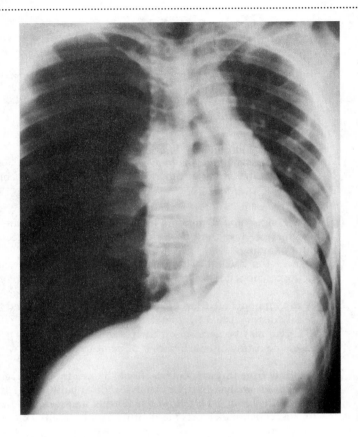

Figure 5-5. Tension pneumothorax in a patient who has penetrating chest trauma. Note the lack of pulmonary vascular markings in the right hemithorax, the mediastinal shift to the left, and depression of the right hemidiaphragm. (Reprinted with permission from Freundlich IM, Bragg DG: A *Radiologic Approach to Diseases of the Chest*, 2nd ed. Baltimore, Williams & Wilkins, p 270.)

(1) **Most common causes** include **chest trauma; emphysema;** and **iatrogenic etiology** (thoracocentesis, transthoracic lung biopsy, mechanical ventilation, central line insertion). Pneumothorax may also be idiopathic.

(2) A **tension pneumothorax** increases in size, which causes a shift of intrathoracic structures.

b. **Clinical features**

(1) Patients report **dyspnea** and **chest pain.**

(2) **Hyperresonance** is detected, and **breath sounds** are decreased over the involved area.

c. **Laboratory findings**

(1) **Chest radiographic films** taken during expiration may more clearly reveal a **pneumothorax,** because they provide more contrast between the lung parenchyma and the air space (Figure 5-5).

(2) **Chest radiographic study** may reveal **mediastinal shift** if tension pneumothorax exists.

d. **Treatment**

(1) A **small pneumothorax** in an asymptomatic patient often requires no therapy.

(2) Pneumothoraces $> 50\%$ usually require treatment.
 (a) **Tube thoracostomy** is the treatment of choice.
 (b) Patients who have a history of recurrence may benefit from **pleurodesis** with intrapleural tetracycline.
(3) Patients who have a **tension pneumothorax** require **immediate therapy with rapid needle thoracentesis** to allow time for the insertion of a chest tube.

3. Pleural neoplasia
 a. General characteristics
  (1) The **most serious** pleural neoplasm is **diffuse malignant mesothelioma.**
  (2) Persons with a **history of asbestos exposure** have an **increased risk of malignant mesothelioma.**
  (3) This neoplasm has a **prolonged latency period** (> 20 years).
 b. **Clinical features** include **chest pain** and **dyspnea.**
 c. Laboratory findings
  (1) **Chest radiographic study** may reveal pleural thickening and/or effusion.
  (2) **Pleural biopsy** is necessary for the diagnosis.
 d. **Treatment** includes **radiotherapy or chemotherapy,** but **response to treatment** is **poor.**

B. Mediastinal diseases

1. Mediastinitis
 a. General characteristics
  (1) **Acute mediastinitis** is **most commonly associated with esophageal perforation** (either from endoscopy or an invading malignancy), **traumatic rupture of the airway, or cardiac surgery.**
  (2) **Chronic disease** is **often secondary to histoplasmosis or sarcoidosis.**
 b. Clinical features
  (1) **Signs and symptoms** include fever, tachycardia, and tachypnea.
  (2) **Pneumomediastinum** may lead to muffled heart sounds, decreased venous return, and subcutaneous emphysema.
  (3) **Pneumothorax** and **pleural effusion** may also occur.
 c. Laboratory findings
  (1) **Chest radiographic study** reveals mediastinal widening, air in the mediastinum and soft tissues, and pneumothorax; fractures of the first three ribs with traumatic bronchial rupture are commonly seen.
  (2) **Leukocytosis** is common.
  (3) **Pleural fluid amylase** levels are elevated, and there is **esophageal rupture.**
 d. Treatment
  (1) Patients should receive appropriate **antibiotics.**
  (2) **Surgical drainage** should be performed.
  (3) The **perforated viscus** should be **surgically closed.**

2. Mediastinal masses
 a. General characteristics
  (1) Most mediastinal masses are **tumors.**
  (2) These tumors may be **benign** or **malignant.**
 b. Clinical features
  (1) **Benign tumors grow slowly** and displace surrounding structures; these tumors are **often painless.**
  (2) **Malignant lesions grow rapidly** and invade and compress structures.
  (3) **Signs and symptoms of malignant lesions** include dysphagia, hoarseness,

stridor, cough, dyspnea, and Horner's syndrome (ptosis, anhydrosis, and miosis ipsilateral to the lesion).

(4) Signs and symptoms of myasthenia gravis may be present in patients who have associated thymoma.

c. Laboratory findings

(1) Chest radiographic study suggests the diagnosis when it reveals the presence of a mass.

(a) Lateral radiographic study is valuable, because masses in the anterior, middle, and posterior mediastinum have differential diagnoses.

(b) Anterior mediastinal masses include thymoma, thyroid mass, germinal cell neoplasms, and lymphoma.

(c) Middle mediastinal masses include bronchogenic cysts, sarcoidosis, and aneurysms.

(d) Posterior mediastinal masses include neurogenic tumors and cysts and esophageal diverticula or neoplasms.

(2) CT scan defines the mass's origin and its relationship to vascular structures more clearly than does radiography.

(3) Biopsy is required for definitive diagnosis of a nonvascular mass.

d. Treatment depends on the etiology of the mass.

C. **Chest wall disorders** are divided into mechanical disorders such as kyphoscoliosis and neuromuscular disorders (see Chapter 7, "Neurologic Diseases").

1. Kyphoscoliosis

a. General characteristics

(1) Posterolateral curvature of the spine → **decreased mobility of chest wall** → **decreased ventilation.**

(2) Kyphoscoliosis occurs **predominantly in women.**

b. Clinical features

(1) Patients experience **exertional dyspnea,** especially if deformity is greater than 70 degrees.

(2) Pulmonary hypertension may develop after prolonged hypoventilation, which leads to right-sided failure.

c. Laboratory findings

(1) Anteroposterior view on **chest radiographic study** reveals curvature of the spine, with crowding of the ribs on the convex side and widened intercostal spaces on the concave side of the curvature; lateral view reveals posterior curvature (Figure 5-6).

(2) Pulmonary function tests are **usually unnecessary** unless a second disorder is suspected.

d. Treatment

(1) Early detection and **therapy during adolescence** can greatly **improve outcome.**

(2) Treatment is administered **when angulation is greater than 40 degrees.**

(3) Patient should wear a **Milwaukee brace** to reduce further curvature.

(4) Surgical correction (Harrington procedure) with spinal fusion and metallic rod insertion may help preserve remaining pulmonary function.

V. NEOPLASMS OF THE LUNG

A. General characteristics

1. Neoplasms of the lung are **often malignant** and may be **primary or metastatic.**

2. These neoplasms are **most commonly associated with a history of cigarette smoking.**

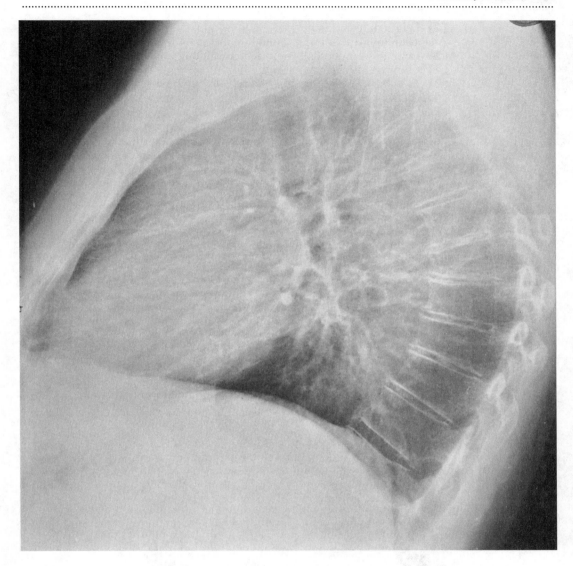

Figure 5-6. Note the extensive curvature of the thoracic spine in this patient who has kyphoscoliosis. (Reprinted with permission from Slaby F, Jacobs ER: NMS *Radiographic Anatomy*. Baltimore, Williams & Wilkins, p 242.)

B. Primary pulmonary neoplasms

    1. General characteristics

        a. Primary pulmonary neoplasms have several **primary histologic variants,** including squamous cell carcinoma, adenocarcinoma, and small-cell (oat) carcinoma.

        b. Squamous cell carcinoma

            (1) Accounts for approximately 40% of all lung cancers

            (2) Is seen in upper lobes and main stem bronchi

            (3) Is a slow-growing tumor

  (4) Is late to metastasize
c. **Adenocarcinoma**
  (1) Accounts for approximately 30% of all lung cancers
  (2) Grows in the peripheral lung
  (3) Is slower growing than squamous cell carcinoma
  (4) Metastasizes early
d. **Small-cell (oat) carcinoma**
  (1) Accounts for 20% of lung cancers
  (2) Has a peripheral origin
  (3) Grows rapidly
  (4) Has usually metastasized at time of diagnosis

2. **Clinical features**
  a. **Signs and symptoms** include weight loss, a cough that has changed in character, dyspnea, and hemoptysis.
  b. A **sign of adenocarcinoma** is **increased sputum** production.
  c. **Digital clubbing** occasionally is seen.
  d. **Pancoast's tumor** is an apical tumor involving the **brachial plexus**; this tumor leads to Horner's syndrome (Figure 5-7).

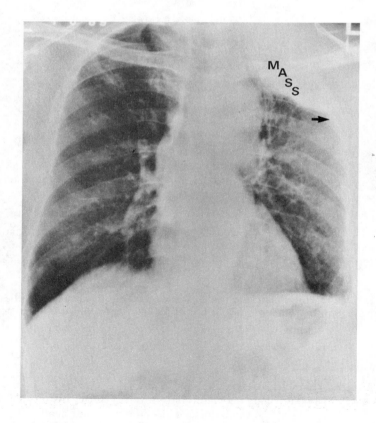

Figure 5-7.   A large left apical mass has destroyed the posterior first to third ribs and merges with the pleura inferiorly. This Pancoast's tumor is formed by a squamous cell carcinoma of the lung. (Reprinted with permission from Freundlich IM, Bragg DG: A *Radiologic Approach to Diseases of the Chest*, 2nd ed. Baltimore, Williams & Wilkins, p 553.)

e. Small-cell tumor is associated with superior vena cava syndrome, which causes facial and upper extremity edema and signs and symptoms of increased intracranial pressure.

f. Wheezing may be present if tumor partially obstructs a bronchus.

g. Recurrent pneumonias are common when a tumor completely obstructs a bronchus.

h. Left hilar mass may involve the left recurrent laryngeal nerve and cause hoarseness.

i. Mediastinal mass may produce diaphragmatic paralysis (phrenic nerve entrapment), which may be detected during physical examination.

j. Common paraneoplastic syndromes seen with pulmonary neoplasm include hypertrophic pulmonary osteoarthropathy, gynecomastia, syndrome of inappropriate antidiuretic hormone, hypercalcemia associated with neoplastic secretion of parathyroid hormone–like substance, and ectopic adrenocorticotropic-producing Cushing's syndrome.

k. Patients may present with metastatic disease rather than pulmonary signs and symptoms; **signs and symptoms of metastatic disease** include:

(1) Enlarged cervical lymph nodes

(2) Bone, pelvis, and back pain due to bony metastasis

(3) Seizure and/or altered mental status due to cerebral metastasis

3. Laboratory findings

a. Sputum cytology is an effective, inexpensive diagnostic test that may reveal the diagnosis if the tumor involves the bronchi; for accurate results, the sputum sample must have a high white blood cell:squamous cell ratio.

b. Chest radiographic study reveals multiple nodules of varying size, or occasionally a solitary pulmonary nodule (see V C); cavitation may be evident.

c. Bronchoscopy is effective in detecting central lesions and should be performed after sputum cytology.

d. Percutaneous needle aspiration with CT guidance is used to obtain samples from small peripheral nodules.

e. Lymph node biopsy is the easiest biopsy technique; in the absence of lymph node involvement, **transbronchial CT-guided or open-lung biopsies** may be necessary.

f. Abnormal liver function results indicate liver metastases; **abnormal bone scan** and **elevated alkaline phosphatase and calcium levels** indicate bone metastases.

4. Treatment

a. Surgical resection is indicated for patients without evidence of metastatic disease.

b. Chemo-/radiotherapy is indicated for small-cell carcinoma.

c. Inadequate FEV_1 precludes surgery (predicted postoperative FEV_1 must be $>$ 0.8 L).

d. Radiotherapy is largely palliative.

C. Solitary pulmonary nodule

1. General characteristics

a. A solitary primary nodule is a **rounded lesion** with **well-demarcated margins.**

b. Between **5% to 40%** of these nodules are **malignant.**

2. Clinical features

a. Patients who have a solitary pulmonary nodule are **usually asymptomatic.**

b. Features associated with benign lesions include:

(1) Diameter $<$ 2 cm

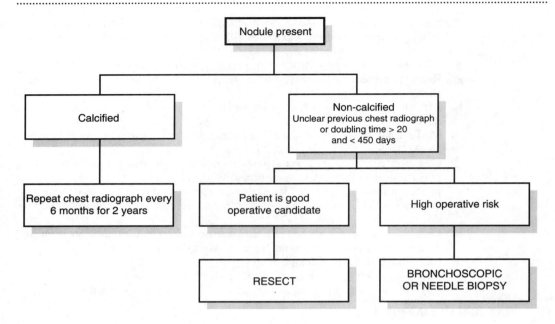

Figure 5-8. Decision algorithm for a pulmonary nodule.

> **(2)** Sharp borders
> **(3)** Non-satellite appearance
> **(4)** "Popcorn" calcification
> **(5)** Age of patient < 40 years

3. Treatment
  a. Because of the potential for malignancy, the physician must **follow up suspicious lesions** (Figure 5-8).
  b. Therapy for malignant lesions includes surgical resection for good operative candidates and **bronchoscopic or needle biopsy** for patients at high operative risk.

VI. PULMONARY DISEASE OF UNKNOWN ETIOLOGY

A. Goodpasture's syndrome

  1. General characteristics
    a. Goodpasture's syndrome is characterized by **intra-alveolar hemorrhage** and **proliferative glomerulonephritis.**
    b. This syndrome **primarily affects men.**
    c. Anti-glomerular basement membrane antibodies also present in this syndrome react with alveolar basement membranes → linear deposition (type II hypersensitivity).

  2. Clinical features
    a. Patients commonly present with **hemoptysis** and **dyspnea.**
    b. Renal failure with azotemia may occur.
    c. Patients may have a **history of respiratory illness** before hemorrhage.

  3. Laboratory findings
  a. **Chest radiographic study** reveals bilateral alveolar infiltrates.
  b. **Pulmonary function tests** indicate a restrictive pattern.
  c. **Iron deficiency anemia** may be present secondary to ongoing pulmonary hemorrhages.
  d. **Serum or tissue (renal or pulmonary) analysis** indicates the presence of anti-glomerular basement membrane antibodies.
  e. **Urinalysis** reveals the presence of red blood cell casts with proteinuria.

  4. Differential diagnosis
  a. **SLE** is distinguished from Goodpasture's syndrome by the lack of anti-glomerular basement membrane antibodies and the presence of antinuclear antibodies and hypocomplementemia.
  b. **Idiopathic pulmonary hemosiderosis** lacks the renal and immune system involvement characteristic of Goodpasture's syndrome.
  c. **Wegener's granulomatosis** is discussed next.

  5. Treatment
  a. **Corticosteroids, immunosuppressive therapy** with alkylating agents, and **plasmapheresis** offer the best results.
  b. **Dialysis** may be required.

B. **Wegener's granulomatosis**

  1. General characteristics
  a. This disease **commonly affects men.**
  b. Wegener's granulomatosis is a **systemic vasculitis** commonly involving the respiratory tract and is **associated with glomerulonephritis.**

  2. Clinical features (see Chapter 1, "Rheumatic Diseases")
  a. **Signs and symptoms** include paranasal sinus pain and drainage, with purulent or bloody nasal discharge.
  b. **Nasal septal perforation with saddle-nose deformity** is often present.
  c. **Additional signs and symptoms** include cough, hemoptysis, dyspnea, and chest discomfort.

  3. Laboratory findings
  a. **Chest radiographic study** reveals the presence of single or multiple focal lesions (unlike the diffuse infiltrates seen in Goodpasture's syndrome).
  b. **Biopsy** is necessary.

  4. Treatment with **cyclophosphamide with or without corticosteroids** produces rapid improvement.

6

Gastrointestinal Disorders

I. DISEASES OF THE ESOPHAGUS AND STOMACH

A. General characteristics

1. These diseases **cause inflammation** and **irritation.**

2. Diseases of the esophagus and stomach include reflux esophagitis, gastritis, neoplasms of the esophagus and stomach, esophageal dysmotility and gastric emptying disorders, and peptic ulcer disease.

B. Reflux esophagitis

1. General characteristics
  a. Reflux esophagitis may be associated with a primary defect in lower esophageal sphincter (LES) tone.
  b. **Secondary causes** include pregnancy; drugs (anticholinergics, β_2-agonists, calcium channel blockers); surgical vagotomy; smoking; and alcohol and caffeine ingestion.

2. Clinical features
  a. **Heartburn** is brought on by bending over or lying down and is associated with a bitter taste in the mouth.
  b. The disease may lead to the formation of **strictures,** which **may cause dysphagia for solid foods.**
  c. **Blood from esophageal erosions** may be present in regurgitated material.
  d. **Signs and symptoms of anemia** may be present if **bleeding** is **chronic or severe.**

3. Laboratory findings
  a. **Barium swallow** and **upper gastrointestinal** (GI) **series test** results are positive only in patients who have severe disease; therefore, these tests are **not very sensitive.**
  b. **Esophageal manometry** allows sensitivity assessment of LES pressures.
  c. **Endoscopy with biopsy** is used to rule out associated peptic ulcer disease and Barrett's esophagus (premalignant epithelial changes associated with chronic reflux).

4. Treatment
  a. **Mild disease** responds to simple measures such as **elevating the head of the bed** and **not eating before bedtime.**
  b. Patients can try **liquid antacids** after meals and before bed.
  c. H_2-**receptor blockers** (cimetidine, ranitidine) are also effective.

d. Antireflux surgery (Nissen fundoplication) should be performed if the patient's disease resists medical therapy.

C. Gastritis

1. Acute gastritis

a. General characteristics

(1) Acute gastritis is defined as a **self-limited inflammation of the gastric mucosa.**

(2) Acute gastritis is commonly **associated with** the use of **acetylsalicylic acid and other** non-steroidal anti-inflammatory drugs **(NSAIDs)**, **ethanol** ingestion, ingestion of **caustic substances,** and **stress.**

b. Clinical features

(1) Common signs and symptoms include dyspepsia, nausea and vomiting, and epigastric pain.

(2) GI bleeding may occur and cause **hematemesis** and **shock,** if severe.

c. Laboratory findings from endoscopic examination are best for diagnosis.

d. Treatment

(1) The patient should refrain from ingestion of the offending agents.

(2) Antacids, sucralfate (a surface-acting agent), and **H$_2$-receptor blockers** lead to rapid healing within days.

(3) Patients who have **severe hemorrhage** respond best to **fluid and blood replacement** and usually do not require surgery.

2. Chronic gastritis

a. Chronic gastritis is **associated with** the use of **NSAIDs, ethanol ingestion, radiation injury,** and **immunologic factors (pernicious anemia).**

b. This disease **lacks definite clinical manifestations** other than anemia associated with atrophic gastritis.

c. Patients who have pernicious anemia lack gastric production of intrinsic factor (IF); the **Schilling test** will therefore be **positive** (i.e., vitamin B$_{12}$ administration alone will not increase urinary vitamin B$_{12}$ excretion, but vitamin B$_{12}$ with IF will increase urinary vitamin B$_{12}$ excretion, which indicates the lack of IF in patients who have pernicious anemia).

d. Patients with chronic gastritis have an increased incidence of gastric ulcer and gastric carcinoma.

e. No specific therapy is indicated **except when pernicious anemia is present,** which requires systemic administration of vitamin B$_{12}$.

D. Neoplasms of the esophagus and stomach

1. Esophageal neoplasms

a. General characteristics

(1) Incidence of esophageal neoplasms is low in the United States.

(2) Esophageal neoplasms **occur most often in men.**

(3) Associated risks include smoking, ethanol ingestion, geographic location (China), lye ingestion, achalasia, and Barrett's esophagus.

b. Clinical features

(1) Patients experience a **progressive dysphagia for solids.**

(2) Signs and symptoms of advanced disease include pain, weight loss, dysphagia for liquids, cough, and hoarseness.

c. Laboratory findings

(1) Barium swallow with a barium-coated bolus is effective in detecting obstruction.

(2) Endoscopy is the **best test** because it allows for biopsy as well as direct visualization of the mass.

(3) **Computed tomography (CT) scan** is useful in assessing spread to adjacent structures.

d. Treatment

(1) **Radiotherapy** is indicated for proximal tumors.

(2) **Surgery** is indicated for middle and distal tumors.

(3) **Stent therapy** may be necessary.

(4) **Survival rates** are **low.**

2. Gastric neoplasms

a. General characteristics

(1) **Incidence** of gastric neoplasms is low in the United States but is considerably higher in Japan.

(2) Gastric neoplasms **occur most frequently in elderly men.**

(3) **Risk factors** include family history, pernicious anemia, previous gastrectomy, and gastric polyps.

(4) These neoplasms **may be due to a gastric lymphoma** resulting from non-Hodgkin's lymphoma.

b. Clinical features

(1) **Signs and symptoms** include weight loss, anorexia, fatigue, epigastric pain, early satiety, and vomiting.

(2) The left supraclavicular node (**Virchow's node**) may be palpable.

c. Laboratory findings

(1) **Upper GI series** is often effective at revealing a mass.

(2) **Endoscopy** is most effective diagnostically and allows for biopsy to establish the diagnosis.

(3) **Elevated serum carcinoembryonic antigen** (CEA) level is a useful biologic marker.

d. Treatment

(1) **Surgical resection** of the affected area is indicated.

(2) **Chemotherapy** may be effective in some patients.

(3) **Surgery and radiotherapy** are indicated for confined gastric lymphoma, with addition of chemotherapy for systemic lymphoma.

E. **Esophageal dysmotility and gastric emptying disorders**

1. Esophageal dysmotility

a. General characteristics

(1) Esophageal dysmotility may be the **result of achalasia** or **diffuse esophageal spasm** (DES).

(2) **Achalasia** results from **absent peristalsis** combined with increased LES tone (Figure 6-1).

(3) This disorder may also be seen in patients who have **scleroderma** (see Chapter 1, "Rheumatic Diseases").

b. Clinical features

(1) **Signs and symptoms** include dysphagia for solids and liquids, chest pain, odynophagia (particularly in diffuse esophageal spasm), and weight loss.

(2) **Achalasia may be associated with nocturnal cough** due to overflow aspiration or with recurrent aspiration pneumonia.

c. Laboratory findings

(1) On a **cine-esophagram,** a dilated **fluid-filled esophagus** (bird-beak) **indicates achalasia; simultaneous, noncoordinated contractions indicate DES.**

(2) **A high LES resting pressure** that fails to relax during swallowing (detected with esophageal manometry) is **associated with achalasia;** the

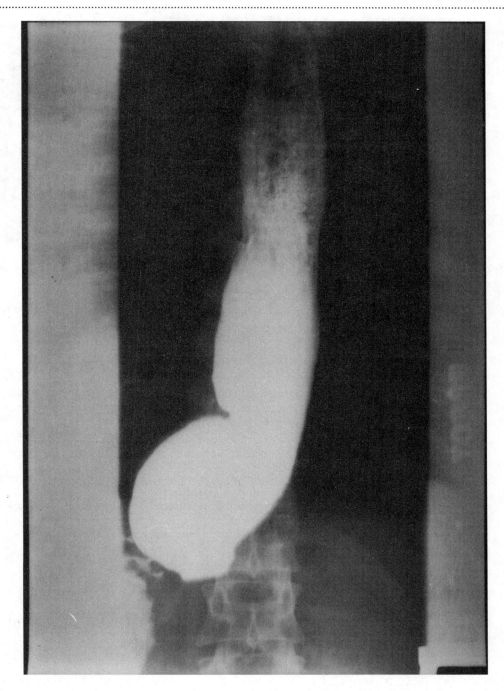

Figure 6-1. Esophagram of a patient who has achalasia. Note the marked esophageal dilatation and narrowing at the gastroesophageal junction due to failure of lower esophageal sphincter relaxation.

presence of **low-amplitude, coordinated contractions** or even the complete **absence of peristalsis distinguishes achalasia from DES.**

   d. Treatment

     (1) For achalasia, **pneumatic dilatation** is often more effective than medical therapy, but this procedure carries a **mortality rate of 0.2% and a perforation rate of 2% to 3%.**

     (2) **Surgical therapy** (Heller's myotomy) for achalasia is also effective but has a **3% to 4% complication rate** as well as a **high risk for the development of postoperative reflux.**

     (3) **For DES,** medical therapy is generally used first and consists of **anticholinergics, nitrates, or calcium channel blockers.**

     (4) **Longitudinal myotomy** is reserved for DES patients who are incapacitated by the disease.

2. Gastric emptying disorders

   a. General characteristics

     (1) Gastric emptying disorders are due to pyloric stenosis, gastric volvulus, gastric bezoars, or gastroparesis.

     (2) **Pyloric stenosis** may be acquired, as in scarring from peptic ulcer disease, or congenital.

     (3) **Gastric volvulus** is often secondary to a paraesophageal hernia.

     (4) **Gastric bezoars** occur in individuals who have had previous gastric surgery or in mentally ill patients who consume indigestible substances such as hair (trichobezoars).

     (5) **Gastroparesis** is most commonly associated with long-standing diabetes.

   b. Clinical features

     (1) **Signs and symptoms of gastric outlet obstruction** predominate, including abdominal pain with minimal distention, nausea, vomiting (which may be projectile), hematemesis, early satiety, and abdominal tenderness and rigidity. **Fever** may be present, particularly when the volvulus is strangulated.

   c. Laboratory findings

     (1) Laboratory findings **vary with the etiology.**

     (2) **Abdominal radiographic study** reveals air in the stomach but little air distal to the obstruction (in **gastroparesis,** air distal to the stomach is observed); two separate left upper quadrant fluid levels may be present in **gastric volvulus.**

     (3) **Endoscopy** may be necessary to rule out malignancy, especially when bezoars are present.

     (4) **Gastric manometry** reveals the presence of gastroparesis.

   d. Treatment

     (1) **Myotomy** is indicated for pyloric stenosis.

     (2) **Bezoars** can be broken down with enzymes or surgically removed.

     (3) **Recurrent nasogastric suction** for volvulus with surgical correction is necessary if vascular compromise is present.

     (4) **Metoclopramide** is indicated for patients who have gastroparesis.

F. Peptic ulcer disease

  1. General characteristics

   a. Peptic ulcers occur in the **stomach** or **proximal duodenum.**

   b. Peptic ulcer disease **occurs most commonly in middle-aged men.**

   c. **Associated risk factors** include smoking, NSAID use, corticosteroid use, ethanol ingestion, family history, and chronic anxiety.

   d. **Duodenal ulcers** are benign, but **gastric ulcers** may be malignant.

pain is most severe in early morning and 2-3 hrs after eating

2. Clinical features   *gnawing pain*
  a. The **main symptom** is an **epigastric burning** sensation.
  b. If the ulcer is **gastric,** the **pain** is **exacerbated by eating;** if duodenal, pain diminishes with eating but occurs 2 to 3 hours after a meal.
  c. Patients may initially be seen with **upper GI hemorrhage,** that is, hematemesis, melena, and abdominal pain.
  d. **Signs and symptoms of anemia** may be present if chronic and/or significant upper GI hemorrhage has occurred.

3. Laboratory findings
  a. **Upper GI series** is more effective in detecting ulcer if performed with **air contrast** and is a useful screening tool, because it is less expensive than endoscopy.
    (1) If no ulcer is found and the clinical suspicion is high, **endoscopy** is still indicated.
    (2) **Features that suggest a benign gastric ulcer** include gastric folds radiating into the base of the ulcer, thick radiolucent edematous collar (Hampton line), smooth crater, and pliable gastric wall in the area of ulcer (Figure 6-2).
  upper endoscopy **b.** **Endoscopy with biopsy** is indicated if initial therapy does not alleviate signs and symptoms or if the clinical situation is highly suggestive of malignant disease.
  c. **Serum gastrin measurements** are rarely indicated unless suspicion of Zollinger-Ellison syndrome (pancreatic gastrinoma leading to recurrent ulcers in distal portions of the duodenum or jejunum) exists.

4. Treatment
  a. **Antacids and H_2-blockers** are equally effective in promoting healing within approximately 4 weeks.
  b. **H_2-blockers** are more convenient than antacids, but cause **side effects** (cimetidine especially) including confusion, tremor and gynecomastia; **ranitidine** is more widely tolerated.
  c. **Sucralfate** is as effective as ranitidine and causes fewer side effects, making this drug **particularly efficacious.**
  d. **Surgery** for intractable cases or complicated peptic ulcer disease is indicated.

II. DISEASES OF THE SMALL INTESTINE

A. Diarrhea
  1. General characteristics
    a. Diarrhea is defined as **increased volume and liquidity of stool.**
    b. **Types** of diarrhea include:
      (1) **Secretory** (caused by *Escherichia coli* toxin, *Salmonella* sp, and *Clostridium perfringens* enterotoxin).
      (2) **Osmotic** (caused by ingestion of nonabsorbable, osmotically active substances such as laxative and lactose in individuals who have lactase deficiency).
    c. **Abnormal intestinal motility** (from rapid or slow peristalsis) causes diarrhea and is most often associated with **long-standing diabetes.**
    d. Long-standing diarrhea may be associated with **irritable bowel syndrome.**
  2. Clinical features
    a. **Persistent diarrhea** in the absence of food intake suggests a **secretory diarrhea.**

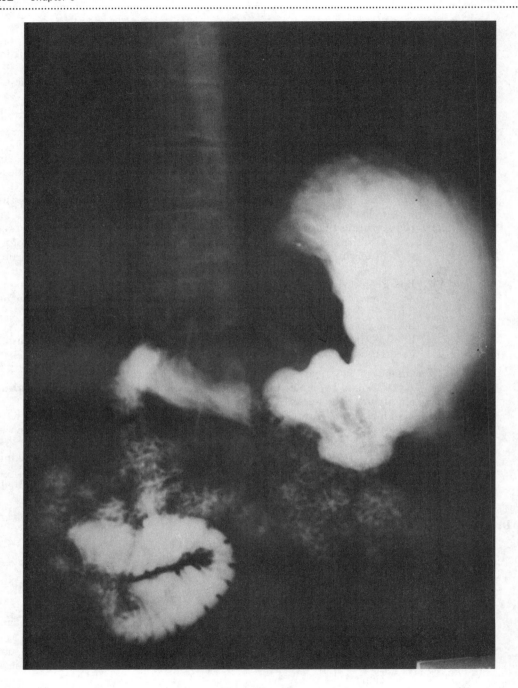

Figure 6-2. Upper gastrointestinal series in a patient who has a benign gastric ulcer. Note the deformity in greater curvature of the antrum. Mucosal folds radiate into the base of the ulcer (an indicator of benignity).

b. Absence of diarrhea after a 2- to 3-day fast suggests **osmotic diarrhea.**

c. Abnormal intestinal motility producing diarrhea may be seen in patients who have **hyperthyroidism or diabetes;** this is largely a diagnosis of exclusion.

d. Alternating diarrhea and constipation with postprandial discomfort and no evidence of nausea, vomiting, weight loss, fever, or GI bleeding suggest **irritable bowel syndrome.**

3. **Laboratory findings**

   a. Stool culture and **sensitivity test** may reveal the presence of a pathogenic bacterial strain.

   b. Microscopic examination of stool may reveal ova or parasites that can cause diarrhea (Table 6-1); often, three samples are sent in order to increase sample yield.

   c. Ion gap calculations can be useful in differentiating secretory from osmotic diarrhea.

   (1) Absence of ion gap between measured stool osmolarity and $2([Na^+] + [K^+])$ present in the stool suggests **secretory diarrhea.**

   (2) The **presence of** such an **ion gap** with an elevated stool osmolarity suggests **osmotic diarrhea.**

Table 6-1
Common Causes of Infectious Diarrhea

Organism	Spread	Comments	Treatment
Escherichia coli	Fecal contamination of food/water	Most common cause of traveler's diarrhea Secretory diarrhea Self-limited	TMP-SMX if severe Pepto-Bismol for symptomatic relief
Campylobacter	Contaminated water or milk	One of the most common causes of bacterial diarrhea in US Self-limited, short duration	Usually not required Ciprofloxacin if prolonged
Salmonella sp	Contamination of eggs or milk	Acute, self-limited Crampy, abdominal pain with fever	Usually no treatment because can lead to prolonged carrier state Severe disease treated with ampicillin or TMP-SMX
Shigella sp	Fecal/oral	Most common in day care centers and urban poor Seen in "gay bowel syndrome" Crampy, abdominal pain progressing to bloody diarrhea if untreated	Ampicillin or TMP-SMX Amoxicillin cannot be substituted because ineffective
Giardia lamblia	Fecal contamination of water	Most common cause of water-borne infectious diarrhea in U.S. Causes mild or severe symptoms	Metronidazole
Norwalk agent/ rotavirus	Person to person	Common cause of self-limited diarrhea	Not necessary

TMP-SMX = trimethoprim-sulfamethoxazole.

    d. **Guaiac test** is used to detect occult blood in the stool.

      (1) Blood in the stool may occur in **invasive infectious diarrhea.**

      (2) Blood in the stool may suggest another pathologic process, such as **inflammatory bowel disease.**

    e. **Wright's or methylene blue staining** of stool detects the presence of white blood cells, which indicate an invasive infectious cause of diarrhea (see Table 6-1).

    f. Figure 6-3 shows the **standard diagnosis algorithm for diarrhea.**

B. **Bacterial food poisoning syndromes** are summarized in Table 6-2.

C. **Small bowel obstruction**

    1. **General characteristics**

      a. Small bowel obstruction may be due to a **mechanical obstruction** such as adhesions from prior surgery or hernia.

      b. Small bowel obstruction can also be **secondary to an adynamic (paralytic) ileus** that can occur with trauma, abdominal surgery, hypokalemia, and peritonitis.

    2. **Clinical features**

      a. **Predominant symptom** is crampy, intermittent abdominal pain.

        (1) The pain is not severe if obstruction is secondary to an adynamic ileus.

        (2) If obstruction is distal, abdominal distention is present.

      b. In a mechanical obstruction, **high-pitched bowel sounds** with peristaltic rushes and tinkles can be heard; **in adynamic ileus, few bowel sounds** can be heard.

      c. **Additional symptoms** include vomiting and constipation.

      d. Obstruction may lead to **intestinal ischemia** and **gangrene.**

    3. **Laboratory findings**

      a. **Abdominal radiographic study** usually establishes the diagnosis.

        (1) **In mechanical obstruction,** characteristic air-fluid levels in distended loops of bowel are evident; air is absent in the rectum.

        (2) **In adynamic ileus,** intestinal gas is diffuse; and air may be present in the rectum.

      b. If **strangulation** and **ischemia** occur, **leukocytosis** may occur.

    4. **Treatment**

      a. **Therapy for adynamic ileus** includes continuous decompression via nasogastric tube and treatment of the primary cause.

      b. **Therapy for mechanical obstruction** includes operative correction if the obstruction is complete and strangulation is in progress; intravenous (IV) hydration, small bowel decompression, correction of electrolyte imbalances, and broad-spectrum antibiotics should be administered before surgery if time permits.

D. **Malabsorption**

    1. **General characteristics**

      a. Malabsorption **may be secondary to a large number of clinical entities.**

      b. **The most common of these entities** include lactase deficiency; inflammatory bowel disease (e.g., Crohn's disease); small bowel infections; chronic pancreatitis (often secondary to alcoholism); obstructive liver disease leading to bile salt deficiency (e.g., cholangiocarcinoma); celiac disease; and long-standing diabetes mellitus.

      c. **Calcium, folic acid, and iron** are absorbed from the proximal small bowel; **bile acids and vitamin B_{12}** are absorbed from the ileum.

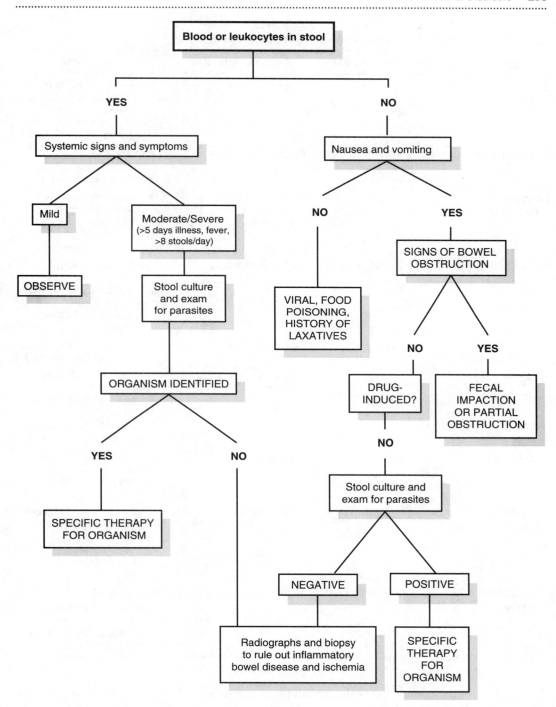

Figure 6-3. Work-up for acute diarrhea.

Table 6-2
Bacterial Food Poisoning Syndromes

Organism	Incubation Period	Source of Infection	Comment
Staphylococcus aureus	2–6 h	Meat and dairy handlers	Sudden onset of vomiting, abdominal pain, and diarrhea Therapy usually not required
Brucella cereus	2–8 h	Reheated fried rice	Vomiting followed by diarrhea Often resolves in 24 h
Clostridium perfringens	8–14 h	Reheated meats, poultry, and legumes	Profuse diarrhea with severe abdominal cramping Rarely lasts > 24 h No therapy required
Salmonella sp	24–48 h	Foods (e.g., eggs)	Diarrhea with low-grade fever Antimicrobial therapy may produce carrier state; therefore, not usually treated
Pathogenic *Escherichia coli*	1–3 d	Food and water	Causes traveler's diarrhea Prophylaxis with TMP-SMX
Vibrio cholerae	1–3 d	Fecally contaminated water	Common in southeast Asia Produces life-threatening diarrhea Treated with intravenous and oral rehydration
Shigella sp	1–3 d	Fecal-oral spread	Diarrhea, fever, bloody stools Treated with ampicillin or TMP-SMX
Clostridium botulinum	1–2 d	Canned foods	Neurologic manifestations Ventilatory support required Requires immediate administration of antitoxin
Clostridium difficile	During or within 4 weeks of discontinuing antibiotic therapy	Antibiotic-associated	Produces pseudomembranous colitis Treated with vancomycin or metronidazole

   d. Absorption of the fat-soluble vitamins A, D, E, and K is impaired when fat absorption is impaired, as can occur in bacterial overgrowth syndrome or pancreatic lipase insufficiency.
2. Clinical features
   a. Features vary with the etiology of the malabsorptive process.

     b. **Signs and symptoms of malabsorption** may include **steatorrhea** (greasy, foul-smelling stools that may float in the toilet bowl); **weight loss; hypoalbuminemia** leading to edema and ascites; and **anemia.**

     c. **Fractures** secondary to poor vitamin D absorption may occur.

     d. **Paresthesias** and **tetany** may result from hypocalcemia.

     e. **Coagulation disorder** may occur due to decreased vitamin K absorption.

  3. Laboratory findings

     a. **Seventy-two-hour fecal fat analysis** is useful in diagnosing malabsorption.

       (1) **Fecal fat more than 6 g/day** indicates **fat malabsorption.**

       (2) **Fecal fat more than 20 to 30 g/day** on a fat diet of 100 g/day is **often associated with pancreatic disease.**

     b. **Decreased absorption** seen **in the xylose absorption test** indicates **injury to intestinal mucosa.**

     c. ^{14}C-xylose conversion to $^{14}CO_2$ is increased in patients who have bacterial overgrowth that can be measured during a breath test.

     d. **Abdominal radiographic study** may reveal a fistula, blind loop, or areas of stasis, which indicate **bacterial overgrowth syndrome.**

     e. **Decreased stool pH** suggests unabsorbed carbohydrates; this sign is **usually seen** in patients who have **lactase deficiency or celiac disease.**

     f. Schilling test (see I C 2 c)

  4. Treatment

     a. Treatment is **based on the underlying cause of the malabsorption.**

     b. **Pancreatic enzyme replacement** is indicated in patients who have **chronic pancreatitis.**

     c. **Ampicillin or tetracycline** may be useful in patients who have **bacterial overgrowth syndrome.**

     d. **Gluten-free diet** should be prescribed for patients who have **celiac disease.**

E. Crohn's disease

  1. General characteristics

     a. Crohn's disease is a **chronic granulomatous disease** that **most often affects the ileum.**

     b. The disease is **often seen** in persons who are **in early adulthood or over age 50.**

     c. **Features** of Crohn's disease include thickened intestinal wall with inflammation, mesenteric lymphadenopathy, ulcerative lesions that may progress to fistula formation, alternating areas of normal and involved bowel wall, and stricture formation secondary to scarring.

  2. Clinical features

     a. **Signs and symptoms** include fever, weight loss, anorexia, colicky pain, and diarrhea.

     b. **A right lower quadrant abdominal mass** may be palpable if the ileum is extensively involved; this sign **mimics appendicitis.**

     c. **Fecal occult blood** is present.

     d. **Colon and rectum involvement** produce significant diarrhea, perirectal fissures, fistulas, and abscesses.

     e. **Peripheral arthritis** may occur in 10% of patients (see Chapter 1, "Rheumatic Diseases").

  3. Laboratory findings

     a. **Abdominal radiographic study** reveals deep ulcerations and long, strictured segments alternating with uninvolved areas (Figure 6-4).

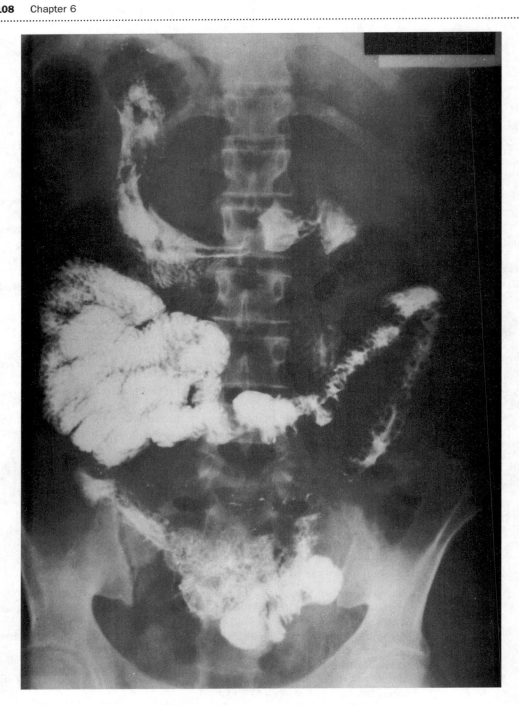

Figure 6-4. Radiographic appearance of Crohn's disease. Swollen folds of mucosa, which are coarse and nodular at the distal jejunum.

b. Endoscopy may reveal inflammatory changes; inflammation can be confirmed with biopsy of affected areas.

c. Anemia, leukocytosis, and protein loss may be present; however, these findings are nonspecific.

4. Treatment

a. In **severe disease, bowel rest** with intravenous (IV) fluid/total parenteral nutrition (TPN) and broad-spectrum antibiotics are indicated.

b. In **acute disease, sulfasalazine therapy** with or without corticosteroids is indicated.

c. Surgery is often required **for fistula formation, abscesses, or obstruction.**

d. Surgical removal of the affected areas is useless because new diseased regions tend to occur proximal to the removed segments; in addition, a significant risk of adhesion and obstruction exists postoperatively.

e. Vitamin B_{12} may be required if the ileum is significantly involved.

III. DISEASES OF THE COLON, RECTUM, AND ANUS

A. General characteristics

1. **The main disorders of the colon** include constipation, appendicitis, diverticular disease, ulcerative colitis, and colonic tumors.

2. **Disorders of the rectum and anus** are largely surgical.

B. Constipation

1. Constipation is defined as **less than three bowel movements per week.**

2. Constipation may be due to a **low-fiber diet** or a **disease process.**

3. **Associated diseases** include ulcerative proctitis, rectal abscess, hypothyroidism, and long-standing diabetes.

4. **Simple constipation** can be treated with increased dietary fruits, vegetables, and bulking agents, whereas **disease-associated constipation** requires treatment of the underlying cause.

C. Appendicitis

1. **General characteristics**

a. Maximum incidence occurs **in the second and third decades of life,** but appendicitis may occur at any time.

b. The disease begins with **obstruction of the appendiceal lumen by a fecalith,** followed by **distention of the appendix** with mucous secretions from the mucosa.

c. Bacterial invasion of the appendiceal wall concomitant with **venous engorgement** and **arterial insufficiency** occur as a result of the increasing intraluminal pressure.

2. **Clinical features**

a. Initially, the patient complains of **periumbilical or epigastric abdominal pain** that may be crampy in nature; **pain eventually localizes** to the right lower quadrant.

b. Nausea and vomiting then develop in 50% to 60% of individuals.

d. Anorexia is extremely common.

e. Tenderness to percussion and palpation in the right lower quadrant (RLQ) is often present.

  f. Rovsing's sign may be present.

  g. If generalized tenderness to palpation and percussion are present, **peritonitis from a ruptured appendix** should be considered.

  h. Positive psoas or obturator signs tend to occur late in the disease process.

  i. Low-grade temperature is **common,** but **temperature greater than 38.3°C** suggests **perforation.**

3. Laboratory findings
  a. Leukocytosis is **common.**
  b. Abdominal radiographs are of little value unless fecalith is demonstrated in the RLQ.
  c. Ultrasound can often confirm the diagnosis when the appendix can be visualized; however, if the appendix cannot be seen by ultrasound, the diagnosis cannot be ruled out.

4. Differential diagnosis includes mittelschmerz (rupture of graafian follicle), mesenteric lymphadenitis, ectopic pregnancy, pelvic inflammatory disease, and Crohn's disease.

5. Treatment
  a. Appendicitis is a **mechanical disease,** and therefore **appendectomy** is the **treatment of choice.**
  b. Intravenous fluids should be administered, because these patients often have had little fluid intake during the onset of the disease.
  c. Antibiotics effective against enteric organisms such as *E. coli* and *Bacteroides fragilis* should be given (e.g., ampicillin/sulbactam) **at the time of diagnosis and** should be **continued postoperatively,** depending upon the presence of perforation.

D. Diverticular disease

1. General characteristics
  a. Diverticular disease is **common in persons older than age 60.**
  b. The disease is **most often found in the sigmoid colon.**
  c. Diverticular disease may be associated with a low-fiber diet.

2. Clinical features
  a. Patients who have this disease are **usually asymptomatic** but may **occasionally have alternating diarrhea** and **constipation** or **crampy abdominal pain** that is relieved by a bowel movement.
  b. Occasionally, **significant painless bleeding from a diverticulum** occurs.
  c. Diverticulitis is a frequent complication.
   (1) Signs and symptoms of diverticulitis include left lower quadrant abdominal pain that worsens with defecation, abdominal tenderness, and fever.
   (2) Inflammatory mass may be palpated in the left lower quadrant.
   (3) Bleeding is usually **microscopic.**

3. Laboratory findings
  a. Plain film abdominal radiographs may suggest the presence of diverticula.
  b. Barium enema is often diagnostic but should not be performed during the acute phase of diverticulitis due to risk of perforation (Figure 6-5).
  c. Sigmoidoscopy/colonoscopy is diagnostic.
  d. Leukocytosis is often present in diverticulitis.

4. Treatment
  a. Increased fiber consumption can relieve some of the uncomfortable symptoms of diverticular disease.

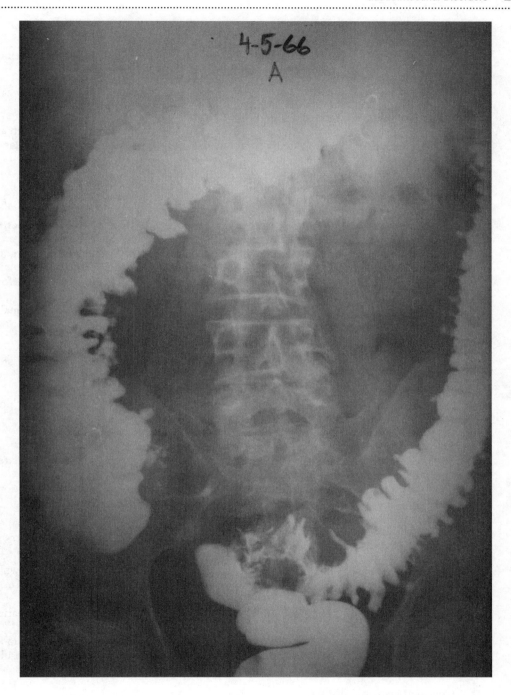

Figure 6-5.   Barium enema in a patient who has diverticular disease of the sigmoid colon. Note the "thumblike" imprints along the wall of the bowel.

    b. Diverticulitis requires **bowel rest** and **broad-spectrum antibiotics.**

    c. **Repeated bouts** of diverticulitis may require **sigmoidectomy.**

    d. **Surgery** may be required if bleeding does not respond to medical management or if fistula or abscess formation occurs.

E. Ulcerative colitis

    1. General characteristics

        a. Ulcerative colitis is characterized by **diffuse inflammation of the rectum and colon;** unlike Crohn's disease, inflamed areas do not alternate with uninflamed area.

        b. Ulcerative colitis is **more common in women than in men.**

        c. **Microabscesses** are produced.

    2. Clinical features

        a. The disease **may be limited to the rectum,** which leads to **ulcerative proctitis.**

        b. **Nocturnal passage of small amounts of blood and mucus** may occur.

        c. **Severe disease** may involve diarrhea, fever, weight loss, abdominal pain, and rectal bleeding.

        d. Severe disease may progress to **toxic megacolon** (Figure 6-6), **colonic perforation, hypokalemia,** and **shock.**

        e. Individuals who have ulcerative colitis are at **increased risk of colonic malignancy.**

    3. Laboratory findings

        a. **Bacterial and parasitic infection** must be ruled out with appropriate stool cultures.

        b. **Malignancy** must be ruled out with colonoscopy and biopsy.

        c. **Analysis of stool sample** reveals presence of blood, mucus, and white blood cells without parasites or bacterial pathogens.

        d. **Barium enema** should not be performed on severely ill patients.

            (1) Barium enema may reveal ulcerations and pseudopolyps.

            (2) This test is an important diagnostic tool that can delineate the extent of bowel involvement.

        e. **Proctoscopy** reveals friable, edematous, hyperemic mucosa with ulcerations.

        f. **Yearly colonoscopic evaluations** are required to rule out neoplastic changes.

    4. Treatment

        a. **Acute flare-ups** can be treated with **bowel rest, IV solutions,** and **TPN,** if necessary.

        b. **Corticosteroids, sulfasalazine,** and **5-aminosalicylate** have been shown to reduce symptoms and induce remission in the acute phase of the disease.

        c. **Sulfasalazine** should be used on a regular basis to prevent recurrence.

        d. **Total colectomy** is required for recurrent, severe disease, or if the patient shows evidence of neoplastic disease.

        e. **Toxic megacolon** requires immediate hospitalization with broad-spectrum antibiotics, replacement of blood and electrolytes, and prompt surgical consultation.

F. Colonic neoplastic disease

    1. General characteristics

        a. Colonic neoplastic disease includes **benign tumors and adenocarcinoma.**

        b. Also included are the **familial polyposis syndromes;** because these syndromes are relatively uncommon, they are not discussed here.

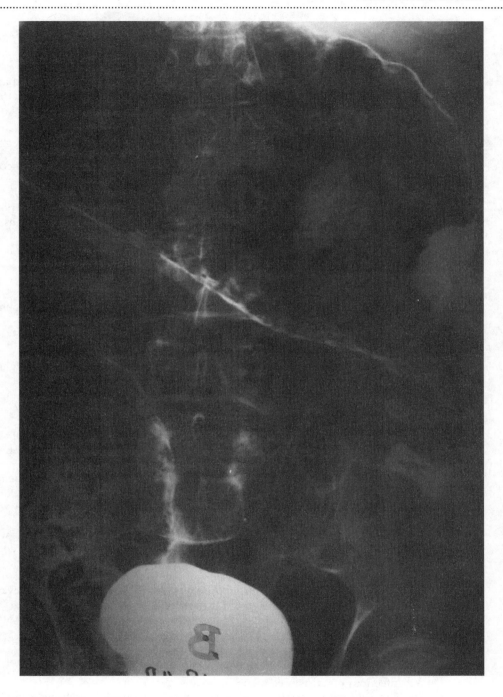

Figure 6-6.   Toxic megacolon. Marked dilatation of the transverse and descending colon is evident in this patient.

2. Benign tumors
   a. General characteristics
   (1) Polyps **may be benign but premalignant.**
   (2) Benign polyps are **commonly found in persons over age 40.**
   (3) **Increased risk of polyp malignancy** is associated with a polyp that is **more than 2 cm** in size, **villous rather than tubular,** and **sessile rather than pedunculated.**
   b. Clinical features
   (1) **Patients who have benign tumors** may be asymptomatic or may have rectal bleeding that can be significant.
   (2) **Patients who have large polyps** may have signs and symptoms of incomplete obstruction.
   c. Laboratory findings
   (1) **Abdominal radiographic study** is usually not diagnostic unless the polyp is large and causes obstruction; however, radiographic study can be useful in excluding diagnoses of GI bleeding.
   (2) **Air-contrast barium enema** is a useful diagnostic tool (Figure 6-7).
   (3) **Endoscopy** is also diagnostic.
   d. Treatment
   (1) **If pedunculated,** the **polyp** may be removed during endoscopy.
   (2) **Other types of polyps** require surgical consultation, because a segmental resection may be required.

3. Adenocarcinoma
   a. General characteristics
   (1) Adenocarcinoma is **one of the most common life-threatening malignancies.**
   (2) Adenocarcinoma is **associated with high red meat and animal fat ingestion.**
   b. Clinical features
   (1) Symptoms include a **change in bowel habits** or a **decrease in stool size.**
   (2) Patients who have **left-sided tumors** often have **obstruction** and/or **hematochezia.**
   (3) Patients who have **right-sided tumors** often have **iron deficiency anemia.**
   c. Laboratory findings
   (1) **Air-contrast barium enema** can delineate the lesion, but **endoscopy with biopsy** is required for diagnosis.
   (2) **Stool analysis for occult blood** should be performed on individuals with suspected disease or for follow-up in patients who have been treated for the disease.
   (3) **Analysis of CEA levels** is not a useful screening tool but can be used for follow-up in patients who have been treated for the disease; **elevated titers** indicate a recurrence or metastasis.
   d. Treatment involves surgical consultation for removal and appropriate postoperative management.

G. Infectious proctitis
   1. General characteristics
   a. Infectious proctitis is **common in homosexual men.**
   b. The disease is **caused by syphilis, gonorrhea, chlamydia,** and **herpes simplex.**
   2. Clinical features
   a. **Tenesmus, constipation, anorectal pain, hematochezia,** and **mucopurulent discharge** may be present.
   b. The **nonspecific signs of fever and leukocytosis** may be present.

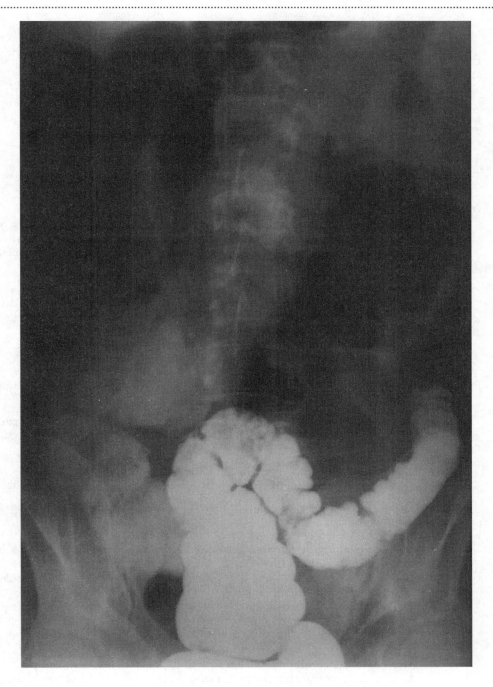

Figure 6-7. Barium enema in a patient who has carcinoma of the descending colon. Numerous loops of distended bowel (small and large) are evident. An annular constricting lesion in the distal portion of the descending colon permits the passage of only a small amount of contrast material to the proximal bowel.

3. Laboratory findings
   a. Culture of sample taken from the anus is **often diagnostic.**
   b. Microscopy of anal sample is **also often diagnostic.**

4. Treatment
   a. **Appropriate antibiotic therapy** is required, for example, penicillin for syphilis and gonorrhea and tetracycline for chlamydia.
   b. **Acyclovir** is indicated for prolonged, frequently recurrent herpes.

IV. PANCREATIC DISORDERS

A. Acute pancreatitis

   1. General characteristics
   a. Acute pancreatitis is defined as **acute inflammation of the pancreas, with edema, autodigestion, necrosis, and hemorrhage.**
   b. **Alcohol ingestion** and **biliary tract disease** are **most commonly associated with pancreatitis.**

   2. Clinical features
   a. Patients experience **steady, severe epigastric pain** that may radiate to the back.
   b. **Nausea and vomiting** usually are not present unless disease is severe.
   c. In severe disease, **abdominal distention** may result from ileus.
   d. Severe disease may lead to **fever, tachycardia, and shock.**
   e. **Epigastric mass** may be **palpable if pseudocyst develops.**
   f. **Hemorrhagic pancreatitis** may cause **Grey Turner's sign** (discoloration of the flanks) or **Cullen's sign** (periumbilical discoloration).

   3. **Differential diagnoses** include biliary colic, perforated viscus (especially if patient has had gastroduodenal ulcers), and acute cholecystitis.

   4. Laboratory findings
   a. **Ultrasound** reveals an enlarged pancreas (also evident on CT scan).
   b. **Diagnosis** is confirmed when positive ultrasound occurs with a significantly elevated serum amylase level (often > 5 times normal).

   5. Treatment
   a. **IV fluid replacement** is required.
   b. **Pain relief** can be achieved **with meperidine** if required; **morphine should be avoided** because it causes spasms of Oddi's sphincter.
   c. **Nasogastric suction** should be performed until the acute phase subsides to allow the pancreas to rest.
   d. **Associated findings** should be treated; for example, hypocalcemia requires calcium, and hyperglycemia requires insulin.

B. Chronic pancreatitis

   1. General characteristics
   a. Chronic pancreatitis is the **progressive destruction and distortion of the pancreas and its ducts.**
   b. The disease is **associated with alcoholism in adults** and **cystic fibrosis in children.**

   2. Clinical features
   a. Patients experience **severe, intractable abdominal pain.**

    b. Eventually, **diabetes and malabsorption with steatorrhea** may occur, which **lead to weight loss.**

    c. **Obstructive jaundice** can occur if fibrous tissue envelops the common bile duct.

    d. **Gastritis** is a **common association,** given its **coexistence with excessive alcohol intake.**

    e. **Hereditary forms** of chronic pancreatitis exist.

3. Differential diagnosis

    a. **Abdominal malignancy** must be considered, especially carcinoma of the pancreas.

    b. **Patients who have peptic ulcer disease** may have **similar presenting symptoms.**

    c. **Biliary tract disease** should also be considered.

4. Laboratory findings

    a. **Analysis of the serum amylase level** is usually not helpful, because the amylase level is elevated in only acute pancreatitis, not chronic disease.

    b. **Abdominal radiographic study** may reveal pancreatic calcification, a cardinal sign of chronic pancreatitis.

    c. **CT scan** may help determine the presence of pancreatic calcification and may also reveal the presence of pseudocysts.

    d. **Endoscopic retrograde cholangiopancreatography (ERCP)** is useful in diagnosing the distorted ductal anatomy.

    e. **Pancreatic stimulation tests** are usually unnecessary but reveal decreased secretion of virtually all pancreatic substances.

5. Treatment

    a. Patients must **reduce alcohol consumption,** if alcohol is a factor.

    b. **Pancreatic digestive enzyme supplements** can be used to reduce the effects of **malabsorption.**

    c. **Insulin** is indicated for **diabetes mellitus.**

    d. **Nonaddictive analgesics** should be used for relief of pain when possible.

C. Pancreatic carcinoma

1. General characteristics

    a. **Smokers and individuals with hereditary forms of pancreatitis** have an **increased risk** of pancreatic carcinoma.

    b. Pancreatic carcinoma has a **high mortality rate.**

    c. The **tumor** is **usually an adenocarcinoma.**

2. Clinical features

    a. **Epigastric pain** and **weight loss** are the cardinal symptoms.

    b. **Pain** is often noncolicky, dull, and persistent.

    c. **Additional signs and symptoms** include anorexia, nausea, vomiting, and diarrhea/steatorrhea.

    d. **Obstructive jaundice** is common when carcinoma affects the head of the pancreas and may lead to a palpable gallbladder.

    e. **Paraneoplastic syndromes** such as Cushing's syndrome or hypercalcemia can occur.

    f. **Invasion of the tumor into the GI tract** may cause upper GI bleeding.

    g. **The diagnosis** should be considered in older patients who have unexplained weight loss, abdominal pain, or recent onset of diabetes without obesity.

3. Laboratory findings

    a. **Presence of tumor markers** (CEA, α-fetoprotein) is generally not useful in diagnosis due to their lack of specificity.

    b. **Ultrasound** and **CT scan** are roughly equal in their efficacy in detecting pancreatic carcinoma.

    c. **ERCP** is often used in conjunction **with the aforementioned imaging techniques** if the diagnosis is uncertain.

    d. **Biopsy with guided aspiration cytology** is required to confirm the diagnosis.

4. Treatment is **mostly palliative** due to the poor response to therapy.

V. BILIARY TRACT DISEASE

  A. Acute cholecystitis

    1. General characteristics

      a. Acute cholecystitis is **defined as an inflammation of the gallbladder.**

      b. It is **most commonly due to obstruction of the cystic duct by an impacted gallstone.**

    2. Clinical features

      a. Patients experience **crampy epigastric or right upper quadrant pain;** pain is **often postprandial** and **subsides in several hours.**

      b. **Fever, nausea, vomiting,** and **ileus** may occur.

      c. **Right upper quadrant tenderness on inspiration** (Murphy's sign) is **common.**

      d. **Jaundice** may be present if the stone impacts the common bile duct.

      e. **Perforation of the gallbladder** may occur, which leads to abscess formation and/or peritonitis.

    3. **Differential diagnoses** include choledocholithiasis, choledochal cysts, and gallbladder or bile duct carcinoma in elderly individuals.

    4. Laboratory findings

      a. Because most gallstones are composed of cholesterol and hence are radiolucent, **abdominal radiographic study** is often of little value.

      b. **Abdominal ultrasound** is useful in detecting gallstones within the gallbladder, but ultrasound cannot detect cystic duct obstruction.

      c. **Radionuclide biliary scan** is the most sensitive diagnostic test because it reveals absence of filling of the gallbladder due to the obstruction.

      d. **Serum analysis** reveals leukocytosis.

    5. Treatment

      a. Patients should receive **IV fluids** and **nasogastric suction** for 24 to 48 hours.

      b. **Surgical removal of the gallbladder when** the **acute phase has subsided** is indicated for patients who are at low operative risk.

      c. **Expectant management** is indicated **for patients who are poor surgical candidates.**

  B. Choledocholithiasis

    1. General characteristics

      a. Choledocholithiasis is defined as the **presence of gallstones in the common bile duct.**

      b. This condition is **most often caused by stones** that have **formed in the gallbladder.**

    2. Clinical features

      a. **Fever, jaundice, and right upper quadrant pain** (Charcot's triad) are the **most common signs and symptoms.**

      b. **Sepsis with cholangitis and shock** may occur in severe disease.

3. Laboratory findings

    a. **Serum analysis** reveals elevated alkaline phosphatase (AP) and transaminase levels.

    b. **Total serum bilirubin** is greater than 85 μmol/L.

    c. **Cholangiography** reveals the obstructed common bile duct.

    d. **Ultrasound of the gallbladder** often reveals the presence of stones, which further supports the diagnosis.

4. Treatment

    a. Patients should receive **antibiotics** (e.g., ampicillin and gentamicin).

    b. Stones can be **removed surgically** or **via endoscopic extraction.**

C. Tumors of the biliary system

    1. General characteristics

        a. **Adenocarcinoma of the gallbladder** is **most common in older women** and is associated with a history of gallstones.

        b. **Adenocarcinoma of the bile duct** is **most common in older men** and is associated with a **history of ulcerative colitis.**

    2. Clinical features

        a. **Signs and symptoms of adenocarcinoma of the gallbladder** mimic those of acute cholecystitis (e.g., right upper quadrant pain); jaundice may be seen if the tumor involves the common bile duct.

        b. **Signs and symptoms of adenocarcinoma of the bile duct** include jaundice with or without pain and weight loss.

    3. Laboratory findings

        a. **Adenocarcinoma of the gallbladder** is **generally diagnosed by the presence of a calcified gallbladder** as revealed by abdominal radiographic study.

        (1) **Histologic examination** confirms the diagnosis.

        (2) **Serum bilirubin levels** do not rise unless the tumor involves the bile ducts and/or liver.

        b. **Adenocarcinoma of the bile duct** is **diagnosed by elevated serum AP** and **bilirubin levels** and only **mild elevations in liver enzyme levels;** diagnosis is confirmed via ERCP with biopsy.

    4. **Treatment** is **palliative,** because the **prognosis** is **poor** for patients who have both tumors.

VI. LIVER DISEASES

A. Viral hepatitis

    1. General characteristics

        a. Viral hepatitis is defined as **a viral, inflammatory disease of the liver.**

        b. Viral hepatitis **may be associated with hepatitis A; B; C (non-A, non-B); or the delta agent** (Table 6-3).

    2. Clinical features

        a. **Signs and symptoms** include malaise, anorexia, fatigue, arthritis, urticaria, and jaundice.

        b. **Influenza-like syndrome** may be present with nausea, vomiting, myalgias, and headache.

        c. **Dark urine/light-colored stools** are caused by impaired bilirubin conjugation.

        d. The **liver is enlarged and tender.**

        e. **Splenomegaly** may occur.

50% hepatitis c pt have cryoglobulinemia (a vasculitic disease caused by Ab that precipitate in cold Tem). Raynaud's phenomenon - livedo reticularis

Table 6-3
Comparison of Viral Hepatitis Agents

Agent	Mechanism of Spread	Incidence with Blood Transfusion	Prevention	Complications
Hepatitis A	Fecal-oral	Rare	Immune serum globulin	Fulminant hepatitis (rarely)
Hepatitis B	Parenteral (e.g., IV drug abusers); sexual contact	10%–20%	Hepatitis B immune globulin; hepatitis B vaccine	Chronic active hepatitis, occasionally causes fulminant hepatitis
Hepatitis C	Parenteral	60%–70%	Immune serum globulin	Same as hepatitis B
Delta agent	Parenteral	Unknown	Unknown	Often present with hepatitis B in cases of fulminant or chronic active hepatitis

3. **Laboratory findings**
   a. Serum aspartate aminotransferase (**AST**) and alanine aminotransferase (**ALT**) levels are **elevated** as much as 20-fold.
   b. AP level is **usually not significantly elevated** (in contrast to biliary disease).
   c. Serum and urine bilirubin levels are increased.
   d. **Serum antibodies and antigens** are **useful diagnostically.**
      (1) **Presence of anti–hepatitis A immunoglobulin M (IgM) antibody** indicates a current or recent infection with hepatitis A within the last 2 to 3 months.
      (2) **Presence of anti–hepatitis A immunoglobulin G (IgG) antibody** indicates prior hepatitis A infection and confers immunity.
      (3) **Presence of** hepatitis B surface antigen (**HB$_s$Ag**) indicates acute or chronic hepatitis B infection.
      (4) **Anti-HB$_s$Ag antibody** is present in late convalescence in acute hepatitis B infection (confers immunity) and is absent in chronic hepatitis.
      (5) **Presence of anti–hepatitis B core antigen (anti-HB$_c$Ag) of the IgM type** indicates current infection with hepatitis B.
      (6) **Presence of** hepatitis B e antigen (**HB$_e$Ag**) without anti-HB$_e$Ag antibody indicates high viral infectivity.
      (7) **Presence of anti–HB$_e$Ag antibody** indicates low infectivity.
      (8) **Presence of anti–hepatitis D antibody** (IgG or IgM) indicates hepatitis D infection.

4. **Treatment**
   a. **No specific therapy** exists.
   b. Patients should maintain **good hydration and dietary intake.**
   c. **Vitamin K administration** may be necessary if coagulation parameters are abnormal.
   d. **Hospitalization** is indicated for patients who have severe nausea/vomiting, prolonged prothrombin time, or severe liver dysfunction.

B. **Alcoholic liver disease**
   1. **General characteristics**

   a. Alcoholic liver disease is seen in the acute stage as **alcoholic fatty liver disease or alcoholic hepatitis.**

   b. Chronic injury results in **alcoholic cirrhosis.**

2. Alcoholic fatty liver disease and alcoholic hepatitis

   a. Clinical features

      (1) Patients who have alcoholic fatty liver disease usually are **asymptomatic,** with **hepatomegaly as the only sign.**

      (2) Fever, jaundice, hepatomegaly, and liver tenderness occur in alcoholic hepatitis.

      (3) Variceal bleeding, encephalopathy, and ascites can be present **in more severe disease.**

   b. Laboratory findings

      (1) Serum γ-glutamyltransferase, AST, ALT, and AP levels are elevated in fatty liver disease.

      (2) Biopsy reveals **large droplet fatty change** in the liver.

      (3) Elevated liver enzymes and bilirubin levels with decreased serum albumin level often **indicate alcoholic hepatitis.**

      (4) Alcohol-induced thrombocytopenia may be present.

      (5) Liver biopsy confirms the diagnosis of **alcoholic hepatitis.**

   c. Treatment

      (1) Patients must maintain **adequate caloric intake.**

      (2) **Thiamine and folate supplements** are required, because these patients are often deficient in these vitamins.

3. Alcoholic cirrhosis

   a. Clinical features

      (1) **Fibrosis** with nodular formation and destruction of normal liver architecture leads to portal hypertension.

      (2) **Initially, the liver** may be **enlarged,** but it **eventually** becomes **small and hard;** a nodular liver may be palpable.

      (3) **Signs of portal hypertension** include ascites, splenomegaly, caput medusae, and variceal bleeding.

      (4) **Liver dysfunction** causes jaundice, spider angiomata, palmar erythema, Dupuytren's contracture, gynecomastia, testicular atrophy, bruising, and fetor hepaticus.

      (5) **Hepatic encephalopathy** occurs with confusion, mood changes, drowsiness, disorientation, and coma.

      (6) **Patients who have hepatorenal syndrome** demonstrate oliguria and progressive renal failure.

   b. Laboratory findings

      (1) **Ultrasound or CT scan** effectively demonstrates the characteristic appearance of the cirrhotic liver.

      (2) **Serum liver enzyme levels** may initially be elevated as dying hepatocytes liberate their enzymes into the blood; as cell death occurs, levels may in fact normalize; **serum albumin level** is often profoundly decreased.

      (3) **Azotemia and electrolyte disturbances** are **common.**

      (4) **In hepatorenal syndrome, elevated blood urea nitrogen and creatinine levels** indicate decreased renal function.

      (5) Prothrombin time is **prolonged.**

   c. Treatment

      (1) **Acute deterioration** requires **hospitalization and management of complications.**

      (2) Patients should consume a **low-protein diet.**

(3) Electrolyte levels must be **stabilized.**

(4) Lactulose decreases nitrogen absorption from the gut.

(5) If necessary, **ascitic fluid** should be **removed in small amounts** due to the risk of hepatorenal syndrome associated with removal of large amounts of fluid.

(6) If **severe bleeding** is present, **clotting factors** should be **administered.**

(7) Variceal bleeding or other types of GI bleeding should be **managed.**

C. Hepatic abscess

1. General characteristics

a. Hepatic abscess **may be due to *Entamoeba histolytica*** (which is seen frequently in homosexual men).

b. Hepatic abscess is **also associated with infection** by the following anaerobes: *E. coli, Klebsiella* sp, *Staphylococcus* sp, and *Streptococcus* sp in conjunction with cholecystitis and cholangitis.

2. Clinical features

a. Signs and symptoms include fever, chills, night sweats, anorexia, liver tenderness, and right upper quadrant pain.

b. Pleuritic pain may also occur.

3. Laboratory findings

a. Blood cultures may be positive for bacteria, which indicates bacteremia.

b. Serum liver enzyme levels are elevated.

c. Serum analysis reveals leukocytosis.

d. Ultrasound and/or CT scan are useful in detecting abscesses greater than 2 cm in size and can also be used to guide needle aspiration for culture and microscopy to confirm the diagnosis.

4. Treatment

a. *E. histolytica* is **treated with amebicides** (e.g., metronidazole) **with aspiration of the abscess.**

b. Broad-spectrum antibiotics (e.g., ampicillin and gentamicin) are **often used to treat bacterial abscesses,** which are commonly polymicrobial; **aspiration of sizable abscesses** is also indicated.

D. Hepatic tumors

1. General characteristics

a. Hepatic tumors consist of both **benign and malignant lesions.**

b. **Benign tumors** are usually of little clinical relevance (unless complicated by hemorrhage).

c. The **liver is one of the most common organ sites for metastatic disease.**

d. The **most common primary malignant tumor is hepatocellular carcinoma** (hepatoma).

2. Hepatoma

a. General characteristics

(1) Hepatoma is **most common in middle-aged men.**

(2) Common associated risks include **cirrhosis** and **prior hepatitis B infection.**

b. Clinical features

(1) Signs and symptoms include malaise, weight loss, abdominal pain, and hepatomegaly.

(2) Hepatic bruit may be audible.

(3) Ascites (may be hemorrhagic) may occur.

(4) **Sudden increase in AP level and acute deterioration in a stable cirrhotic patient** are hallmarks of hepatoma.

c. **Laboratory findings**

(1) **Serum AP level is elevated,** with a less significant increase in liver transaminase levels.

(2) **Alpha-fetoprotein** level is **often elevated.**

(3) **Angiography** reveals a **hypervascular mass within the liver.**

(4) **Liver biopsy** must be performed cautiously because of the vascular nature of the tumor.

d. **Treatment**

(1) **No successful treatment** exists.

(2) **Prognosis** is **poor.**

7
Neurologic Diseases

I. CEREBROVASCULAR DISEASE

A. Stroke

1. **General characteristics**
   a. May be **ischemic** (arterial thrombosis, venous thrombosis, and arterial embolism) or **hemorrhagic** (intracerebral hemorrhage or subarachnoid hemorrhage) (Figure 7-1).
   b. A stroke can cause **permanent or temporary neurologic deficits.**
      (1) Patient may have a permanent neurologic deficit.
      (2) Patient may have **transient ischemic attacks** (TIA, defined as a neurologic deficit that persists for less than 24 hours).
      (3) Patient may have a **reversible ischemic neurologic deficit** (RIND, defined as a neurologic deficit that slowly resolves over days to weeks).
   c. **Stroke incidence** increases with age.
   d. **Risk factors** are divided into **major** and **minor contributors** (Table 7-1).
   e. **Lacunar strokes** are **caused by occlusion of** small, penetrating **intracerebral arteries** and are **most commonly associated with hypertension** or **diabetes mellitus.**

2. **Clinical features**
   a. Any of the following **signs and symptoms** may be present: sudden onset of neurologic deficit, headache, loss of consciousness, speech disturbance such as dysarthria and aphasia, homonymous hemifield visual deficits, and contralateral motor and/or sensory deficits.
   b. **Signs and symptoms associated with the brain stem or cerebellum** include dysarthria, dysphagia, ataxia, diplopia, vertigo, nausea, nystagmus, ipsilateral numbness, and contralateral motor deficits.
   c. **Infarcts involving the middle cerebral artery** can result in aphasia if the dominant hemisphere is affected, along with contralateral muscle weakness that is more pronounced in the face and arm than in the leg.
   d. **Infarcts involving the anterior cerebral artery distribution** typically cause more significant weakness in the contralateral leg than in the contralateral arm and face.
   e. **Infarcts involving the contralateral posterior cerebral artery distribution** typically cause an isolated homonymous hemianopia.
   f. **Transient monocular blindness** indicates involvement of the carotid system (as opposed to the vertebrobasilar system); **monocular blindness** is often caused by an embolus from a carotid plaque that occludes the retinal artery.

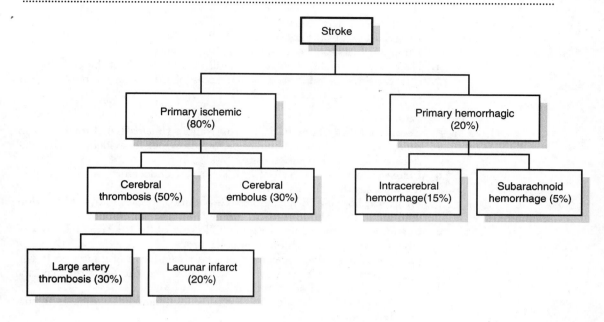

Figure 7-1.   The majority of strokes are secondary to an ischemic event; for example, they are associated with a thrombus or embolic phenomenon rather than a primary hemorrhagic event.

g. A **pure motor stroke** usually results from a small infarct in the posterior limb of the internal capsule that causes equal one-sided loss of face, arm, and leg strength (no sensory loss or cortical dysfunction).

h. **Bilateral visual loss** suggests ischemia of the vertebrobasilar system.

i. **Patients who have an intracerebral hemorrhage** may or may not experience acute onset of severe headache; if the hemorrhage is severe, the patient may develop signs and symptoms of increased intracranial pressure, including vomiting, decreased level of consciousness, pupillary asymmetry, and posturing of the extremities.

Table 7-1
Risk Factors for Stroke

Major	Minor
Age	Hypercholesterolemia
Male gender	Obesity
Race (African-American)	Physical inactivity
Family history	Oral contraceptive use
Diabetes	Alcohol consumption
Smoking	
Hypertension	
Prior stroke	
TIAs	
Cardiac disease (e.g., atrial fibrillation with thrombus)	
Asymptomatic bruit	

TIA = treatment ischemic attack.

    j. **Carotid bruit** may be detected.

    k. **Irregular heart beat** suggests atrial fibrillation, which can result in thrombus formation that leads to a cerebral embolic event.

    l. **Heart murmurs** may suggest endocarditis as the origin of the embolus.

    m. The **presence of multiple vascular areas of infarction** strongly suggests cerebral embolus (multiple emboli).

  3. Laboratory findings

    a. **Complete blood count (CBC), prothrombin time/partial thromboplastin time,** and **platelet count** should be performed to look for evidence of coagulation problems and hyperviscosity.

    b. **Increased white blood cells (WBCs)** suggest endocarditis as the cause of the embolus that leads to stroke.

    c. **Electrocardiogram (ECG)** should be obtained, because atrial fibrillation with mural thrombus formation can be the origin for emboli.

    d. **Results of a computed tomographic (CT) scan of the head** can differentiate a hemorrhagic from a thromboembolic stroke.

      (1) **Lacunar strokes** typically appear as a small area of infarction in the subcortical area (usually < 1 cm); however, the CT scan may not reveal any area of infarction.

      (2) An **initially ischemic area** that **becomes hemorrhagic** suggests an embolic etiology.

      (3) The presence of **intraventricular blood** is **associated with a hemorrhagic stroke** and a **poor prognosis.**

    e. **Serum cholesterol level** may be elevated and **suggests a stenotic artery** as the origin of the thromboembolus.

    f. **Doppler studies of the carotid arteries** are often warranted in a patient who has TIAs originating from the carotid artery circulation; these studies are effective in detecting stenotic vessels.

    g. **Lumbar puncture** is **not routinely indicated and, in fact, is contraindicated** due to the risk of herniation in patients who have mass effects associated with the stroke; **indications for lumbar puncture** include suspected syphilis, meningeal irritation, or an unexplained fever.

    h. **Blood cultures** should be performed **if bacterial endocarditis is suspected** or **if the patient has an unexplained fever.**

    i. **Magnetic resonance imaging (MRI)** is not required in the initial evaluation of a patient who has stroke, because the **CT scan effectively distinguishes hemorrhagic stroke from a thromboembolic stroke.**

  4. Treatment

    a. **Patients who have lacunar strokes** typically have a **good prognosis for recovery.**

      (1) Patients require **hypertension and diabetic control** (if applicable).

      (2) Patients also require **intensive rehabilitation therapy.**

    b. **Early, vigorous treatment of hypertension** immediately **after a non-hemorrhagic stroke** is **not indicated** because hypotension may lead to further ischemic insult; **gradual lowering** of the **blood pressure is desirable** unless the patient is in hypertensive crisis.

    c. **Anticoagulation therapy** (e.g., sodium warfarin) is **indicated for a cardiogenic source of emboli** if the stroke is non-hemorrhagic.

    d. **Patients who experience TIAs** or **are at increased risk for stroke** may take daily doses of aspirin.

    e. For hemorrhagic stroke, **mannitol, intubation with hyperventilation,** and

nystagmus with a strictly vertical direction is usually related to a central lesion in the pons or medulla.

elevation of the head of the bed may be warranted if the patient has **signs and symptoms of increased intracranial pressure.**

(1) **Aggressive control of elevated blood pressure** also decreases elevated intracranial pressure.

(2) **Cerebellar hematomas** are **particularly responsive to surgical evacuation** if they are surgically accessible.

B. Subarachnoid hemorrhage

1. General characteristics

a. The **most common non-traumatic causes** of **subarachnoid hemorrhage** include ruptured intracranial aneurysm and bleeding of an arteriovenous malformation (AVM).

b. AVMs usually occur in persons under the age of 40; AVMs **are congenital** and **twice as common in men.**

c. **Intracranial aneurysms** may bleed at any time but **are more likely to bleed during periods of stress with increased blood pressure;** intracranial aneurysms are **usually congenital.**

2. Clinical features

a. Patients experience acute onset of **severe, localized headache.**

b. **Meningismus** may be present.

c. **Focal neurologic deficits** may or may not be present.

d. **Seizure** may be the first sign of an AVM.

3. Laboratory findings

a. **CBC** and **coagulation studies** should be performed to assess **the patient's coagulation ability,** because **surgical intervention** is often immediately necessary.

b. **Cerebral angiography** remains **diagnostic for** both **AVM and cerebral aneurysm; cerebral artery vasospasm** may become evident 2 to 3 days following a bleed.

c. **Initial CT scan** should be performed in order to localize the lesion and confirm or rule out the presence of subarachnoid/intracerebral blood.

4. Treatment

a. **Neurosurgical consultation** is necessary.

b. **Appropriate antiseizure therapy** should be administered if the patient has seizure; therapy includes **diazepam** and **ventilatory support,** if needed.

c. **Increased intracranial pressure** should be managed, for example, with elevation of the head of the bed, mannitol, intubation, and hyperventilation.

II. DISORDERS OF HIGHER COGNITIVE FUNCTION

A. General characteristics

1. Lesions in specific cortical areas of the brain produce recognizable clinical symptoms.

2. Lesions of the frontal, parietal, temporal, and occipital lobes as well as anterior, posterior, and conductive aphasia are discussed here.

B. Frontal lobe lesions

1. General characteristics

a. Frontal lobe contusions often result from head injury.

    b. These **lesions may be infarcted** by anterior communicating artery aneurysm rupture or compressed by a meningioma arising from the olfactory groove.

    c. Patients exhibit **lack of social appropriateness and inhibitions,** which may lead to urination or masturbation in public.

    d. **Perseveration** is present.

    e. **Stroking the hand** from lateral to medial aspect leads to the **sustained grasping reflex.**

    f. **Stroking the thenar eminence** leads to **twitching of the ipsilateral corner of the mouth** (palmo-mental reflex).

C. Temporal lobe lesions

  1. General characteristics

    a. Temporal lobe lesions **often produce seizures.**

    b. **Aphasia** may occur if the lesion progresses posteriorly on the dominant hemisphere.

    c. **Superior quadrantic hemianopia** occurs when Meyer's loop is involved.

  2. Clinical features

    a. Patients exhibit **brief, repetitive behaviors** (e.g., lip-smacking, eye-twitching, chewing).

    b. **Seizures are preceded by an aura** that may be olfactory or gustatory.

    c. Patients may experience an **intense feeling of unfamiliarity or familiarity with their surroundings.**

    d. Patients **appear to be in a daze** and **rarely lose consciousness.**

D. Occipital lobe lesions

  1. **Bilateral occipital lobe involvement** produces cortical blindness in which the pupillary response (which involves brain stem nuclei only) is maintained, but vision is lost.

  2. A **single affected occipital lobe** leads to a crossed homonymous hemianopia.

  3. **Occipital lobe lesions** may occur secondary to basilar artery occlusion.

E. Parietal lobe lesions

  1. Parietal lobe lesions are **characterized by a visual field attention deficit in the contralateral visual field;** a left-sided parietal lobe lesion produces an inability to see movement of fingers in the patient's right visual field when fingers in both visual fields are moved.

  2. Patients exhibit **contralateral astereognosis** (inability to recognize objects by feeling their shape) and **neglect of contralateral body parts.**

  3. If the lesion is present on the dominant side, **finger agnosia** may be present (inability to name fingers).

  4. **Lower homonymous hemianopia** may occur.

  5. **Acalculia** may be present.

F. Aphasia

  1. Expressive aphasia (Broca's aphasia)

    a. **Spontaneous language production** is slow.

    b. Patients **often overuse and repeat nouns.**

    c. **Little intonation** is present in speech.

    d. **Comprehension of language** is good.

    e. **Proximity of the lesion to the facial motor strip** may lead to associated contralateral facial palsy.

    f. **Patients often appear distressed about the inability to clearly express themselves** because they comprehend their disability.

2. Receptive aphasia (Wernicke's aphasia)

    a. Patients can **generate speech, but it contains few nouns** and **lacks meaning.**

    b. Patients may use **unknown meaningless words** (neologisms).

    c. **Comprehension** is **impaired.**

    d. Patients often have **poor insight into** their **deficit.**

3. Conduction aphasia

    a. Patients' speech contains **semantic confusions.**

    b. Patients exhibit **little dysphasia** and **good comprehension.**

    c. Patients have **poor ability to repeat heard words.**

III. DEMENTIA

A. General characteristics

1. Dementia is an **acquired, persistent, and progressive impairment of intellectual function.**

2. Dementia **may cause compromise in language, memory, visuospatial skills, or cognition** (calculation, abstraction, judgment).

3. Sixty percent to seventy percent of senile dementia cases are **due to Alzheimer's disease;** 15% to 20% are **multi-infarct dementias.**

4. Multi-infarct dementia is **more common in men** and is **associated with hypertension.**

    a. **Drugs** that commonly cause dementia include sedatives, ranitidine and cimetidine, neuroleptics, anticholinergics, and nonsteroidal anti-inflammatory drugs (NSAIDs).

    b. **Chronic alcohol abuse** can also produce signs and symptoms of dementia.

2. Clinical features

    a. **Signs and symptoms of dementia** include:

      (1) Forgetfulness in the absence of depression

      (2) Loss of computational ability

      (3) Word-finding and concentration problems (e.g., inability to read a paragraph)

      (4) Difficulties with daily activities, such as dressing or balancing a checkbook

      (5) Progression to severe memory loss, disorientation, and social withdrawal.

    b. **Patients who have Alzheimer's disease** experience an **insidious onset** and **steady progression of signs and symptoms.**

    c. **Patients who have multi-infarct dementia** exhibit a **stepwise deterioration.**

    d. **Rapid onset and short duration of dementia** suggest a **treatable cause** such as infection or drug-associated dementia.

    e. **Normal-pressure hydrocephalus is associated with** the triad of **dementia urinary incontinence,** and **gait instability.**

    f. **Depression** can be **mistaken for dementia.**

      (1) These patients also **perform poorly on mental status examinations,** may be **irritable,** and exhibit **short attention spans.**

(2) The **depressed patient** is more likely to complain about difficulty answering mental status examination questions, whereas the **demented patient** is usually oblivious to his/her errors.

3. Laboratory findings
   a. Analysis of serum electrolyte, glucose, calcium, thyroid-stimulating hormone (TSH), and vitamin B_{12} levels should be performed to exclude curable causes.
   b. **Elevated cholesterol level** may be seen in patients who have **multi-infarct dementia** (non-specific).
   c. If **hypoxemia** is suspected, an **arterial blood gas analysis** should be performed to confirm the presence of this condition.
   d. **Urinalysis** should also be performed, because an ongoing urinary tract infection can produce symptoms of dementia.
   e. If it is difficult to **differentiate between multi-infarct dementia and Alzheimer's disease** from history and physical examination, a **CT scan or MRI** can detect the presence of multi-infarct dementia; no clear changes on CT scan or MRI are associated with Alzheimer's disease.

4. Treatment
   a. **Reversible causes** should be treated; for example, discontinue any suspected medications known to have a side effect of dementia; correct any electrolyte, mineral, and/or vitamin deficiencies; and treat any apparent infections.
   b. If **no reversible cause** is found, and **Alzheimer's disease** is **strongly suspected,** a small percentage of patients have shown **improvement with** the use of **tacrine; occupational therapy** and **social services** help the patient and family cope with this disease.
   c. **Cessation of smoking** and **treatment of hypertension** may alter the natural course of multi-infarct dementia.
   d. **Treatment of depression** (psychiatric referral) should be initiated if the diagnosis is established.

IV. SEIZURE DISORDERS

A. General characteristics

1. Seizures may be caused by:
   a. **Metabolic disorders** (e.g., hypocalcemia, hypoglycemia, alcohol withdrawal)
   b. **Trauma** (usually manifests within 2 years after a head injury)
   c. **Tumors** (especially if the seizure occurs after age 30)
   d. **Cerebrovascular disease most commonly causes seizures after age 60**
   e. **Infectious disease**
      (1) History of **supratentorial brain abscess** carries a high risk of seizures.
      (2) **Infectious causes** must be ruled out if the physical examination reveals **signs and symptoms of meningitis or cerebral abscess.**

2. Seizures may also be **idiopathic** or **congenital.**

3. **Types of seizures** include simple partial, complex partial, generalized, and febrile.
   a. In **simple partial seizures,** no loss or disturbance in consciousness occurs; seizure activity depends on the portion of the brain affected (e.g., a motor seizure involving the left leg indicates seizure activity originating in the right cortical motor strip associated with leg function).

     b. **Complex partial seizures** resemble simple partial seizures except that an associated disturbance or loss of consciousness occurs.

     c. **Generalized seizures** may be absence seizures (i.e., petit mal); myoclonic; or tonic-clonic (grand mal).

        (1) Generalized seizures are **associated with loss of consciousness or loss of responsiveness/awareness;** no focal origin is suggested by the seizure's appearance (i.e., the seizure involves the entire body rather than initiating in one particular limb).

        (2) Generalized seizures **may arise from a partial seizure;** a generalized seizure may begin in, for example, the arm and then become generalized over the entire body.

        (3) **Urinary/fecal incontinence** may occur.

        (4) **Confusion, fatigue, headache, and disorientation** may occur **after** the seizure (postictal state).

        (5) These **seizures** may be **unrelenting** (status epilepticus).

     d. **Febrile seizures typically occur between ages 18 months and 5 years.**

        (1) Febrile seizures can occur in normally healthy children.

        (2) These seizures usually last no longer than a few moments and occur after a rise in body temperature.

B. **Clinical features**

    1. **No relationship** typically exists **between postural changes** and the **onset of seizures** (compared with vasovagal syncope).

    2. The **neurologic examination** is **often normal** in patients who have seizures; the **exception** is the **patient who has sustained developmental delay from recurrent seizures during infancy.**

    3. **Lateralizing signs** may be seen immediately **following focal seizures** that may **point out** the **affected area.**

    4. **Temporal lobe seizures** are often preceded by an **aura** (often of an odor or a feeling of strange, intense familiarity with the surroundings).

    5. **Petit mal seizures** typically last less than 15 seconds.

    6. It is important to **differentiate seizure from syncope** (a patient experiencing syncope usually does not bite the tongue, which is commonly seen in generalized seizures).

    7. **Pseudoseizures** are seizure-like episodes of psychogenic origin.

     a. Pseudoseizures can be **distinguished from true seizure disorders** by variations in the seizure types described by the patient and by the clinician's observation of a tight association between seizures and stressors or significant personal events.

     b. Patients who have pseudoseizures may report an **awareness of their surroundings during a "grand-mal" seizure** (this awareness does not occur in a true grand-mal seizure).

C. **Laboratory findings**

    1. **CT scan/MRI** should be ordered for patients who have seizures of focal origin (i.e., partial seizures) and for patients more than 30 years of age with new onset of seizures, because these individuals may have an **underlying neoplasm.**

    2. **Electroencephalogram (EEG)** may be helpful in classifying the seizure disorder and thereby assist in guiding therapy; EEG may be useful intraoperatively when removing epileptogenic foci.

Table 7-2

Commonly Used Anticonvulsants

Seizure Type	Drug
Grand mal and/or partial	Phenytoin
	Carbamazepine
	Valproic acid
Petit mal	Ethosuximide
	Valproic acid
Myoclonic	Valproic acid

3. **CBC, glucose, and renal and liver function tests** should be performed if the patient is older than age 10 in order to **rule out metabolic causes** as well as **provide a baseline for organ function monitoring** and **side effects of anticonvulsants.**

D. Treatment

1. Patients should be **referred to a neurologist.**

2. Patients are treated with **anticonvulsive therapy** appropriate to the seizure type (Table 7-2).

3. If the **maximum dose of one anticonvulsant** has been reached, but **no improvement** is noted in the seizure disorder, then a **second anticonvulsant** may be added to the regimen while the first drug is tapered.

4. **Plasma drug levels** must be monitored in order to ensure compliance and adequate dosing regimens.

5. **Status epilepticus** is managed with maintenance of the airway; **25 to 50 mL of 50% dextrose** are administered if **hypoglycemia** is the cause. **Intravenous diazepam 10 mg** are given over 2 minutes if the patient does not improve; a **repeat dose** is given in 10 minutes if the patient still does not improve.

6. **Children who have febrile convulsions** should receive **0.5 mg/kg of diazepam** administered rectally.

V. HEADACHES

A. General characteristics

1. Headaches may be **chronic or acute.**

2. **Acute onset** of headache in a patient previously healthy **suggests an organic cause.**

3. **Headache types** include classic migraine, common migraine, tension headache, cluster headache, trigeminal neuralgia, and giant cell arteritis.

B. Clinical features

1. **Classic migraine** is associated with a **prodromal aura,** which is usually a transient visual, motor, or sensory phenomenon.
   a. Headache is **typically unilateral** and **pulsating.**
   b. Headache is **preceded by a prodrome.**
   c. Headache may **persist** for 1 to 2 days.

    d. Pain may vary from **mild to severe.**

    e. Some **prodromal symptoms** may be severe and produce transient hemiplegia, aphasia, or hemisensory deficits.

2. **Common migraine** is not associated with a prodromal aura.

    a. Pain is **unilateral or bilateral** and is **usually intense.**

    b. Pain usually affects the **eyes, frontal regions, and temples.**

    c. Headache typically **lasts for a day or longer.**

    d. Both types of **migraines tend to begin in adolescence or early adulthood** and may be associated with **vomiting.**

3. **Tension headache** is characterized by a feeling of tightness, pressure, and constriction.

    a. These headaches are **often associated with stressors.**

    b. Pain is **commonly suboccipital** and **nonthrobbing.**

    c. Tension headaches may be **associated with prolonged positioning of** the **head** and neck.

4. **Cluster headaches** recur over periods of **weeks to months, followed by** periods with **no headache.**

    a. Cluster headaches are **most common in middle-aged men with leonine facies** and a **history of heavy smoking or drinking.**

    b. Each headache typically lasts **30 minutes to 2 hours.**

    c. Pain is **unilateral** and occurs **around** the eye.

    d. **Horner's syndrome** may be present.

    e. Headache may be associated with **nasal congestion/rhinorrhea.**

    f. Pain radiates to the **ipsilateral neck or jaw.**

    g. **Ipsilateral conjunctival injection** and **ipsilateral facial redness** may be seen.

    h. Alcohol is a common **trigger.**

5. **Trigeminal neuralgia** appears in the **middle to later part of life** and is **more common in women.**

    a. Trigeminal neuralgia is characterized by momentary, **sudden, lancinating facial pain.**

    b. Pain typically arises **on one side of the mouth** and then **radiates** to the eye, ear, and/or nostril on the ipsilateral side.

    c. Pain may be **precipitated by touch, movement, breezes,** or **eating.**

    d. **Attacks tend to increase in frequency.**

    e. **Neurologic examination** is **usually normal** unless an underlying disease is present (e.g., multiple sclerosis).

6. **Giant cell** (temporal) **arteritis** (see Chapter 1 VIII H) is another type of headache.

C. Laboratory findings

    1. **If a patient has neurologic findings, behavioral changes, or a chronic persistent headache,** then **WBC count, TSH/thyroxine analysis, CT scan,** and **EEG** should be ordered to **rule out** a possible infectious, hormonal, or **cerebral tumor etiology.**   MS

    2. In a **young patient who has trigeminal neuralgia, multiple sclerosis** must be suspected; **cerebrospinal fluid (CSF)** and **nerve conduction studies** may corroborate this suspicion (see multiple sclerosis, XI).

    3. **CT scan** may be necessary to rule out posterior fossa tumor.

D. Treatment

1. **Migraine** treatment consists of:
   a. **Resting** in a **quiet, dark room**
   b. Initial treatment with **aspirin**
   c. Ergotamine and caffeine combination
   d. **Sumatriptan** (a drug with an affinity for serotonin receptors)
      (1) Sumatriptan is injected subcutaneously and is effective in many patients who are refractory to the aforementioned therapies
      (2) This drug is contraindicated in pregnant patients
   e. **Prophylactic treatment** if patients experience migraines more than two to three times a month (e.g., amitriptyline)
   f. **Calcium channel blockers** (e.g., nifedipine)

2. **Cluster headache** treatment consists of:
   a. **Inhalation of 100% oxygen** for 15 minutes
   b. **Ergotamine tartrate aerosol** (may be given prophylactically as well)
   c. **Amitriptyline** for prophylaxis

3. **Trigeminal neuralgia** treatment consists of:
   a. **Carbamazepine** (most often effective)
   b. **Neurosurgery consultation** if patients are refractory to therapy
      (1) A significant number of refractory patients may have an **impinging vascular structure** adjacent to the trigeminal nerve root
      (2) **Multiple sclerosis** must be excluded

4. **Tension headache** treatment consists of:
   a. **Stress relief exercises**
   b. **Aspirin** or **acetaminophen**
   c. **Antimigrainous agents** if patient is refractory to simple analgesics

5. **For treatment of giant cell arteritis,** see Chapter 1, "Rheumatic Diseases," VIII H 4.

VI. MOVEMENT DISORDERS

A. Benign essential tremor

1. **General characteristics**
   a. Benign essential tremors **commonly occur after age 40;** incidence increases with age.
   b. These tremors may **be familial related.**
   c. Diagnosis should be **distinguished from Parkinson's disease** (see VI B).

2. **Clinical features**
   a. **Postural tremor** is often seen in the hands.
   b. **Tremor attenuates with movement** but becomes more obvious when the target is reached (e.g., when a patient attempts to grab a glass, the tremor is initially minimal but becomes more pronounced just before picking up the glass).
   c. **Frequency of the tremor** is typically between 7 and 11 cycles per second (c/s).

3. **Laboratory findings** are **typically not used in the diagnosis,** which is most often made by history and physical examination.

4. Treatment
   a. **One or two ounces of alcohol** may improve the tremor.
   b. If tremor is disabling, **propranolol or primidone** may be effective in reducing the severity.

B. **Parkinson's disease**

   1. General characteristics
      a. Parkinson's disease is the **most frequently encountered extrapyramidal movement disorder.**
      b. This neurodegenerative disease **begins most often in the fifth and sixth decades** of life.
      c. Parkinson's disease is **characterized by low dopamine levels in the corpus striatum.** *especially substantia niagra*

   2. Clinical features
      a. Patients exhibit a **resting tremor** that **usually is initially seen in one extremity.**
         (1) **Frequency of the tremor is typically 4 to 7 c/s.**
         (2) Tremor may be **pill-rolling** in nature.
         (3) Tremor **decreases with movement of** the **affected limb.**
      b. Patients have **difficulty buttoning shirts** and **dressing** and **cutting food;** alterations in **handwriting** are noted.
      c. Patients report a feeling of **stiffness** and **overall slowness** in movement **(bradykinesia).**
      d. **Rising from** a **low sitting position** is difficult.
      e. Patients exhibit **propulsion** (inability to stop walking forward).
      f. **Masked facies** is present.
      g. **Posture** is **stooped** and **flexed.**
      h. **Cogwheel rigidity** may be present unilaterally or bilaterally.
      i. Patients have **impaired postural reflexes** (seen when a patient turns around and must take several small shuffling steps in order to maintain balance).
      j. The **duration and rate of onset of signs and symptoms** is **important,** because Parkinson's disease is a **slow, progressive disease** that develops over months to years; **acute onset** of parkinsonian symptoms **suggests intoxication** (e.g., carbon monoxide).

   3. Laboratory findings
      a. **Diagnosis** is based on **history and physical examination.**
      b. **CT scan of the head** may be used to rule out other diagnostic possibilities such as normal pressure hydrocephalus.
      c. **Apomorphine** (a short-acting dopamine agonist) can be used as a therapeutic challenge; if symptoms improve, Parkinson's disease is confirmed.

   4. Treatment   *Lewy body (eosinophilic intranuclear inclusion body)*
      a. **No cure** exists.
      b. **Amantadine** is often used for patients who have mild symptoms.
      c. **Anticholinergic drugs** (e.g., benztropine) tend to alleviate tremor and rigidity rather than bradykinesia; these drugs are **contraindicated** in patients who have **narrow-angle glaucoma.**
      d. Levodopa (a drug that is converted into dopamine in situ) **alleviates the signs and symptoms but does not stop the progression** of the disease.
         (1) **Dyskinesia,** a major side effect, necessitates "drug holidays."
         (2) **Patient response to levodopa is unpredictable.**
         (3) **Carbidopa** is an inhibitor of the enzyme that breaks down peripheral

dopamine in the body; therefore, it is **used to decrease** the **dose of dopamine** administered.

    e. **Bromocriptine** acts on dopamine receptors and can be used synergistically with **levodopa/carbidopa.**

C. **Huntington's disease**

    1. General characteristics

        a. Huntington's disease is characterized by **chorea** and **dementia.**

        b. The disease is **autosomal dominant.**

        c. Onset is delayed until **after age 30** (usually after the patient has had children).

        d. The disease is caused by decreased **gamma-aminobutyric acid** and cholinergic activity relative to dopamine activity.

    2. Clinical features

        a. Huntington's disease is **progressive,** with a **fatal outcome** within 15 to 20 years.

        b. **Early changes** include irritability, moodiness, and antisocial behavior.

        c. **Subsequent dementia** occurs.

        d. **Dyskinesia** may begin as restlessness and progress to choreiform movements.

        e. Patients exhibit **irregular, involuntary hand and facial movements.**

        f. **Reflexes** are typically brisk.

        g. **Smooth eye pursuit movements** are absent.

        h. **Stance** is wide with variable cadence.

        i. Patients are unable to maintain **tongue protrusion.**

    3. Laboratory findings

        a. **Diagnosis** is based on history and physical examination.

        b. **Recombinant deoxyribonucleic acid testing** is used to diagnose family members of patients with Huntington's disease (particularly children of affected individuals); test is 99% accurate.

    4. Treatment

        a. **No cure** exists.

        b. **Dopamine-blocking agents** such as phenothiazines or haloperidol may control dyskinesia and behavioral problems.

        c. **Reserpine,** which blocks neurotransmitter reuptake and therefore depletes stores of dopamine, has provided some benefit.

        d. **Genetic counseling** is recommended for children of patients.

D. **Tourette's syndrome**

    1. General characteristics

        a. **Signs and symptoms** begin **before age 15.**

        b. Tourette's syndrome is a **chronic, lifelong disorder** with relapses and remissions.

    2. Clinical features

        a. **Motor tics** are usually the first sign; tics commonly involve the face and may include sniffing, blinking, or frowning.

        b. Phonic tics may also occur.

             (1) **Phonic tics** consist of barking, grunting, throat-clearing, or coughing.

             (2) **Coprolalia** (obscene speech) or **echolalia** (repeating the speech of others) may be present.

    3. **Laboratory findings** are **usually unnecessary** because the diagnosis is based on history and physical examination.

4. Treatment
- **a.** Clonazepam and clonidine are used as first-line drugs.
- **b.** Haloperidol is effective but has extrapyramidal side effects.
- **c.** Pimozide (dopamine antagonist) may be useful in individuals who cannot tolerate or are unresponsive to haloperidol.

E. Wilson's disease

1. General characteristics
- **a.** Wilson's disease is **characterized by hepatolenticular degeneration.**
- **b.** The disease is **rare autosomal recessive.**
- **c.** Onset occurs **between the first and third decades of life.**
- **d.** **Excessive deposition of copper in the liver and brain** is an important feature of this disease.
  - **(1)** Excess copper deposition is caused by increased absorption of copper from the bowel and decreased excretion by the liver.
  - **(2)** This feature is important because it is a reversible cause of neurologic and hepatic dysfunction.

2. Clinical features
- **a.** Patients may exhibit **rigidity** and **parkinsonian tremor.**
- **b.** **Dysarthria** is a consistent finding.
- **c.** **Neurologic symptoms** progress slowly over years.
- **d.** **Psychiatric disorders** may be present and vary from adjustment disorder to depression to schizophrenia.
- **e.** **Kayser-Fleischer rings** (fine, pigmented, brownish deposits in the cornea) may be present.
- **f.** **Hepatitis** is often the earliest sign of the disease (occurring before the neurologic signs and symptoms).
  - **(1)** **Patients with hepatitis have jaundice, malaise, and anorexia,** which **usually** spontaneously **resolve.**
  - **(2)** **Cirrhosis** may be detected.

3. Laboratory findings
- **a.** **Urine copper level** is >100 $\mu g/24$ h.
- **b.** **Ceruloplasmin level** is decreased (<20 $\mu g/dL$).

4. Treatment
- **a.** **Early treatment** is necessary to prevent permanent hepatic and neurologic damage.
- **b.** **Penicillamine** enhances urinary excretion of chelated copper.
- **c.** **Pyridoxine** is given in conjunction **with penicillamine** treatment because penicillamine is a pyridoxine antimetabolite.
- **d.** Patients should **restrict** their **intake of dietary copper** (shellfish, legumes).
- **e.** **Oral zinc** decreases gastrointestinal absorption of copper and may be used as maintenance therapy.
- **f.** **Screening tests for family members** of affected individuals are recommended.

VII. SPINAL CORD SYNDROMES

A. Traumatic injury to the spinal cord

1. General characteristics
- **a.** Traumatic spinal cord injuries **usually occur** in the **prime of life.**

    b. These injuries are **commonly associated** with **motor vehicle accidents, diving accidents,** and **falls.**

  2. Clinical features

    a. If conscious, the patient reports a **lack of feeling and paralysis below** the level of the **injury.**

    b. If the patient is unconscious, a spinal cord injury must be assumed; **care** must be taken when **placing** this patient in a **cervical spinal collar.**

    c. The **cervical, thoracic,** and/or **lumbar spines** are often **tender to palpation when a vertebra** is **fractured.**

    d. **Reflexes** may be brisk below the level of the lesion.

  3. Laboratory findings

    a. **Anterior, lateral, and open mouth radiographic views** should be obtained in any patient suspected of having a spinal cord injury; if necessary, **flexion, extension, and a swimmer's view** should also be obtained.

    b. If clinical suspicion exists, and radiographs are equivocal, **CT scan or MRI** can be used to assess for cervical spine fracture.

    c. If clinical suspicion is high for a spinal cord injury, but radiographs are unrevealing, **immobilization** must be continued until the presence or absence of neurologic injury can be confirmed clinically.

  4. Treatment

    a. **Spinal immobilization** must be maintained.

    b. **Neurosurgical consultation** is necessary.

    c. **Methylprednisolone** may be of benefit if given within 8 hours of the injury.

    d. **Long-term management** requires transfer to a center equipped to care for spinal cord injury patients.

B. Cervical spinal and radicular syndromes

  1. General characteristics

    a. **Whiplash injury** is a **common cause** of these syndromes.

    b. **Spondylotic degenerative cervical spine changes** are another common cause.

  2. Clinical features

    a. **Whiplash usually** occurs during a **motor vehicle accident commonly involving** a **rear-end collision.**

      (1) Patient is **usually in the vehicle** and is **wearing a seat belt.**

      (2) Commonly, **neck pain** begins a **few hours after the injury,** although it is not uncommon for neck pain to begin immediately after the collision.

      (3) Pain is **exacerbated by movement.**

      (4) Pain may be **accompanied by occipital headache.**

      (5) **Severe injury,** especially in individuals with preexisting spondylotic degenerative disease, **may produce cervical radicular syndromes** (see following text).

    b. **Spondylotic degenerative changes most commonly affect C6–C7.**

    c. In C-6 injury:

      (1) **Deep, boring pain** is **referred** to the **upper arm and shoulder.**

      (2) **Pain** is exaggerated with neck movement.

      (3) **Tingling and numbness** occur in the index finger and thumb.

      (4) **Biceps reflex** is depressed.

      (5) **Biceps and brachioradialis muscles** weaken (weak supination and flexion at the elbow).

     d. In C-7 injury:

       (1) **Pain** is **referred** to the arm and forearm.

       (2) **Sensory disturbance** occurs in the middle finger.

       (3) **Triceps reflex** is depressed and weakened.

3. Laboratory findings

    a. In patients who have spondolytic degenerative changes, **radiographic study** may reveal osteophyte formation and narrowing of the intervertebral disk space.

    b. **MRI** is particularly effective in detecting disk propulsion into the spinal cord.

    c. **Whiplash injury typically** does not appear **in radiographic studies because** it **typically involves** the **ligaments.**

4. Treatment

    a. A **soft collar** may provide some comfort.

    b. **Analgesics** such as NSAIDs may be of benefit.

    c. **Continued pain and weakness** may necessitate a **neurosurgical decompression** of the affected nerve root.

C. Lumbar spinal and radicular syndromes

  1. General characteristics

    a. These syndromes are **most often due to prolapsed intervertebral lumbar disks.**

    b. Patients may have a **history of awkward lifting or straining.**

    c. **Injury most commonly arises at the L5–S1 level** (70%), which causes compression of the first sacral root, followed by injury at L4–L5 (25%), which causes compression of the fifth lumbar root.

  2. Clinical features

    a. Patients experience **sciatica, or pain in the buttock** and down the back of the thigh and leg.

    b. **S-1 compression** causes **tingling** along the outer aspect of the foot, with **numbness** corresponding over the S-1 dermatome (Figure 7-2).

      (1) **Ankle tendon reflex** is decreased.

      (2) If compression is severe, the **gastrocnemius muscle may begin to atrophy.**

    c. **L-5 compression** causes weakness of the extensor hallucis longus (extension of the great toe), with varying degrees of footdrop; sensory deficit occurs along the outer aspect of the leg and dorsum of the foot.

  3. Laboratory findings

    a. **Radiographs** may reveal narrowing of lumbar disk spaces.

    b. **MRI** may show herniated disk material and a compressed nerve root.

    c. These studies are necessary if the patient requires surgery (i.e., the patient does not respond to conservative management).

  4. Treatment

    a. **Conservative management** includes bed rest and NSAIDs.

    b. **Steroid injections** are not beneficial.

    c. **Surgical consultation** is necessary if signs and symptoms do not subside after 2 to 4 weeks of conservative management and radiography reveals evidence of nerve root compression.

D. Extramedullary lesions

  1. General characteristics

    a. **Lesions occur outside the dura** but cause signs and symptoms due to spinal cord compression.

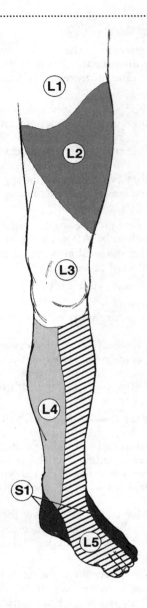

Figure 7-2. Dermatomes of the leg. L2—gray shading, L3—clear, L4—dotted, L5—lined, S1—black.

    b. The lesions may be caused by metastatic spread of a tumor to vertebral bodies (e.g., breast, lung, or prostatic metastasis); **vertebral infection** (e.g., tuberculosis); or **extradural hematoma** (associated with anticoagulant therapy).

    c. Primary tumors such as meningiomas and neurofibromas (more common than intramedullary tumors) **may also cause cord compression.**

2. Clinical features

    a. Presence of fever suggests infectious etiology.

b. **History of prostatic, breast, or lung cancer** should prompt a search for bony metastasis.

c. **Radicular pain** is felt at the dermatomal level of the lesion.

d. **Ipsilateral extremity weakness and sensory deficits** eventually progress to the contralateral extremity as the lesion expands.

e. Patients may experience **urgency of micturition and impotency.**

f. **Cauda equina syndrome** occurs if a lesion compresses the sacral and lumbar roots as these roots stream caudally (e.g., central L4–L5 disk herniation).

    (1) This compression causes **loss of sphincter control.**

    (2) Patients experience **numbness in the buttocks and the back of the thighs.**

    (3) **Weakness/paralysis of dorsiflexion of the foot (L4) and toes** (L4–L5) and **plantar flexion** (S1) occur.

3. **Laboratory findings**

    a. **Radiographs** may reveal calcification associated with a tumor mass.

    b. **CT scan and MRI** are often more revealing of the nature and extent of the lesion.

    c. **Bone scans** are often performed on patients who have prostatic or breast carcinoma in order to rule out bony metastases.

4. **Treatment**

    a. If the lesion is caused by an infection, the **abscess must be surgically drained,** and the **patient** should be **started on appropriate antibiotic therapy** (e.g., isoniazid for tuberculosis).

    b. **Neurosurgical consultation** is necessary.

E. **Intramedullary lesions**

  1. **General characteristics**

    a. These **lesions** occur **within the spinal cord.**

    b. **Types of intramedullary lesions** include astrocytomas, ependymomas, syringomyelia, vascular infarcts, or plaque demyelination in association with multiple sclerosis.

  2. **Clinical features**

    a. **Syringomyelia or a centrally located ependymoma** impairs pain and temperature sensation and spares pinprick sensation and proprioception (dissociated sensory loss); **sacral sparing is typical** (this sign differentiates an intramedullary lesion from an extramedullary lesion).

    b. **A lesion involving the left portion of the spinal cord** causes ipsilateral weakness and contralateral lack of pain and temperature sensation below the lesion.

  3. **Laboratory findings**

    a. **CT scan and MRI** are required for delineation of the lesion.

    b. **CSF** may reveal presence of malignant cells.

  4. **Treatment** requires a neurosurgical consultation regarding surgical resectability versus chemotherapy/radiotherapy.

VIII. NEUROCUTANEOUS SYNDROMES

A. **Tuberous sclerosis**

  1. **General characteristics**

    a. This disease may be **sporadic or autosomal dominant with variable penetrance.**

    b. Tuberous sclerosis is a **multiple intracerebral hamartoma.**

2. **Clinical features**
   a. Patients are **initially** seen in early childhood to have **seizures** and **psychomotor retardation.**
   b. **Reddened nodules on the face** appear **between ages 5 and 10.**
   c. **CT scan/MRI** reveals the intracranial lesions.

3. **Treatment**
   a. **No specific treatment** is available.
   b. **Anticonvulsant drugs** may control seizures.

B. **Neurofibromatosis**

1. **General characteristics**
   a. The disease may be **sporadic** or **autosomal dominant with variable penetrance.**
   b. Two types exist:
      (1) **Type I (Recklinghausen's disease)** is characterized by multiple hyperpigmented macules and neurofibromas.
      (2) **Type II** is characterized by intraspinal, intracranial tumors and a high incidence of multiple, bilateral, acoustic neuromas.

2. **Clinical features**
   a. **Café au lait spots** (patches of cutaneous pigmentation) appear.
   b. **CT scan/MRI** is used for diagnosis and to follow up on the growth of lesions.

3. **Treatment** involves **surgical resection of symptomatic tumors.**

C. **Sturge-Weber syndrome**

1. **General characteristics:** This **congenital syndrome** is caused by a **unilateral cutaneous capillary angioma** involving the **upper face** and **leading to leptomeningeal angiomatosis.**

2. **Clinical features**
   a. Patients may have **focal or generalized seizures** secondary to the leptomeningeal angiomatosis.
   b. **Contralateral hemiparesis and hemisensory disturbance** may be present.
   c. **Radiographs** taken after age 2 usually reveal **gyriform intracranial calcification** in the parieto-occipital region beneath the intracranial angioma.

3. **Treatment**
   a. Treatment is aimed at **controlling seizures pharmacologically** (see seizure disorders, IV).
   b. If seizures are refractory to medical therapy, **surgical excision** may be necessary.

IX. PERIPHERAL NEURAL DISORDERS

A. **Polyneuropathies**

1. **General characteristics**
   a. **Subacute polyneuropathy** may occur secondary to a primary process, such as diabetes mellitus, chronic renal failure, deficiency in vitamin B_{12}, and alcoholism.
   b. **Polyneuropathy** may occur as a primary process (e.g., Guillain-Barré syndrome).

2. Clinical features

    a. Patients have **unpleasant paresthesias** (prickling or burning sensations) **in the tips of the toes** or on the **soles of feet.**

    b. Paresthesias may then **spread to fingertips.**

    c. **Muscle weakness** is usually not prominent if the onset of the disease is slow.

    d. **Ankle and knee jerks** are decreased.

    e. Patients **lose vibration sensation** before losing light touch sensation.

    f. **Positive Romberg's sign** and **ataxia** may be present.

    g. **Guillain-Barré syndrome** is characterized by an ascending paralysis.

        (1) This syndrome occurs **at any age.**

        (2) It is **often preceded by a viral prodrome.**

        (3) Patients have **weak, rubbery, painful legs.**

        (4) **Ascending weakness** with **quadriparesis** and **ventilatory insufficiency** may ensue within 48 hours or develop over a period of up to 3 weeks.

        (5) **Cranial nerve VII** is **often affected,** causing **bilateral facial motor weakness.**

3. Laboratory findings

    a. **Evaluation** is primarily based on **patient history and physical examination** in order to narrow the diagnostic possibilities.

    b. **Elevated blood sugar level** suggests a diabetic etiology.

    c. **Elevated blood alcohol level and decreased serum vitamin B$_{12}$ level** often coexist in alcoholics.

    d. **Elevated serum creatinine and blood urea nitrogen levels** exist in individuals who have chronic renal failure.

    e. **CSF analysis** reveals an elevated protein level and often a normal or increased lymphocyte count in Guillain-Barré syndrome.

4. Treatment

    a. Treatment is **based on etiology.**

    b. **Progression of diabetic neuropathy** can be decreased with strict diabetic control; pain often spontaneously resolves after a period of a year.

    c. **Vitamin B$_{12}$ deficiency** is treated with replacement of the vitamin through regular injections or oral supplements.

    d. **Guillain-Barré syndrome** is managed with respiratory support.

        (1) The **disease spontaneously resolves.**

        (2) **Plasmapheresis** may hasten recovery if performed within 7 days of onset of the disease.

B. Mononeuropathies

1. Carpal tunnel syndrome

    a. General characteristics

        (1) Carpal tunnel syndrome is **caused by compression of the median nerve beneath the carpal ligament** secondary to synovitis of the tendon sheaths or a poorly healed fracture.

        (2) Carpal tunnel syndrome may also be **caused by repetitive use of the hands** (often seen in typists).

    b. Clinical features

        (1) Patients experience **burning and tingling** in the lateral aspect of the hand (first three fingers) along the palmar aspect and the dorsal aspect of the second and third fingers distal to the middle interphalangeal joint (Figure 7-3).

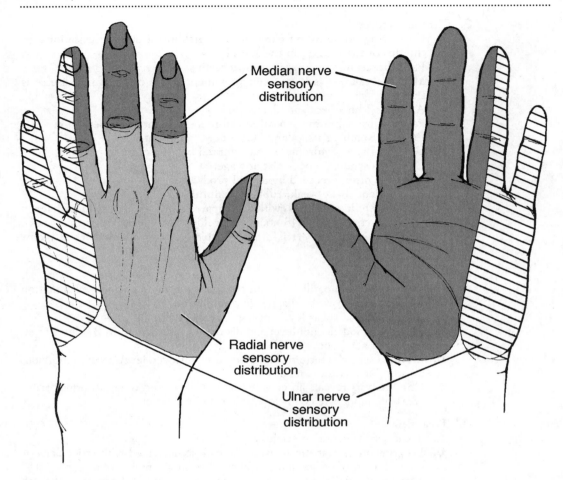

Figure 7-3.   Cutaneous innervation of the hand. Dark gray—median sensory distribution, light gray—radial nerve sensory distribution; hatched—ulnar nerve sensory distribution.

       (2) **Pain may radiate into the forearm** and is exacerbated by manual activity, especially with flexion and extension of the wrist.

       (3) **Sensation** is **impaired** in the median nerve distribution.

       (4) **Tinel's sign** may be positive (pain on percussion of the volar aspect of the wrist).

       (5) **Abductor pollicis brevis atrophy** occurs later.

       (6) **Electromyography** (EMG) may show conduction delay in the median nerve.

    c. Treatment

       (1) **Splinting of the hand and forearm** may sufficiently reduce signs and symptoms.

       (2) Individuals who have **synovitis of the wrist** may benefit from **steroid injection** into the carpal tunnel.

       (3) **Refractory or severely affected individuals** should undergo **surgical division of the carpal tunnel ligament.**

2. Radial nerve injury
   a. The radial nerve is **commonly injured at the axilla** due to the pressure of crutches or when the arm hangs over the back of a chair.
   b. The **injured nerve causes weakness or paralysis of the arm extension** at the elbow, wrist extension, metacarpophalangeal joint extension, and thumb extension.
   c. A **secondary sensory deficit** may occur at the dorsolateral aspect of the hand (see Figure 7-3).

3. Ulnar nerve injury
   a. **Trauma or pressure typically occurs behind the medial epicondyle** (may be seen in persons undergoing surgery who have been improperly positioned).
   b. **Sensory changes** occur in the medial 1.5 fingers and along the medial border of the hand (see Figure 7-3).
   c. **Wrist inversion** (flexor carpi ulnaris function), **palmar abduction,** and **thumb adduction** may be weak.

4. Sciatic nerve palsy
   a. Sciatic nerve palsy is **commonly caused by a misplaced intramuscular injection** in the buttock **or trauma to the buttock or** hip area.
   b. **Weakness of dorsiflexion and eversion of the foot** are present.
   c. **Sensory deficit** occurs along the anterolateral aspect of the calf and dorsum of the foot.

5. Bell's facial palsy
   a. General characteristics
      (1) Bell's facial palsy is an **idiopathic facial paresis** and **may be associated with herpes simplex virus.**
      (2) This palsy **affects the lower motor neuron** and lasts a few days.
   b. Clinical features
      (1) Patients experience a **sudden onset of paresis** that is **often accompanied by ear pain.**
      (2) Patients are **unable to completely close the ipsilateral eye.**
      (3) **Disturbance of taste** due to involvement of chorda tympani fibers may also be present.
   c. Treatment
      (1) **Sixty percent** of patients **recover** completely **without treatment.**
      (2) Individuals who have a **complete palsy** are **less likely to fully recover** and require treatment.
      (3) **Recommended treatment** is **oral prednisone** for 4 to 5 days, followed by a tapering dose.
      (4) If **eye closure** is affected, **lubricating eyedrops** and an **eye patch** may be helpful.
      (5) **Surgical procedures** to decompress the facial nerve have not proved to be beneficial.

X. NEUROMUSCULAR DISORDERS

   A. Amyotrophic lateral sclerosis (ALS)

      1. General characteristics
         a. ALS is a **degeneration of anterior horn cells** (lower motoneurons) and **pyramidal neurons** (upper motoneurons).
         b. Most cases occur sporadically.
         c. The **cause** of ALS remains **unknown.**

2. Clinical features
   a. Patients experience **asymmetric weakness and atrophy.**
   b. **Footdrop** and/or **clawhand deformity** are common.
   c. **Fasciculations** and/or **spasticity** may be seen.
   d. **Hyperreflexia** in an atrophic fasciculating extremity strongly suggests the diagnosis.
   e. **Spread to virtually all muscle groups** may occur over weeks to months.
   f. **Facial and eye movements** tend to be spared.
   g. Most patients succumb to **respiratory insufficiency or infection** within 2 to 3 years.

3. Laboratory findings
   a. **EMG** is most diagnostic because it reveals abnormal spontaneous activity in resting muscles.
   b. **Sensory conduction studies** are normal.
   c. **CSF** is normal.
   d. **Serum creatine kinase level** may be slightly elevated but not to the degree seen in muscular dystrophies.

4. Treatment
   a. Treatment is **symptomatic.**
   b. **Stretching exercises** prevent contractures.
   c. **Adaptive equipment and bracing** are required.
   d. **Swallowing dysfunction** may lead to aspiration or choking; the patient must be closely watched.
   e. **Diazepam** may relieve a degree of spasticity.

B. Myasthenia gravis

1. General characteristics
   a. Myasthenia gravis **may occur at any age.**
   b. This disease can be **associated with thymic tumors or thyrotoxicosis.**
   c. Disease occurs **most commonly in young women with HLA-DR3.**
   d. **Onset** is **usually insidious,** but may be unmasked by a coincidental infection that exacerbates symptoms.
   e. The disease has an **autoimmune etiology.**

2. Clinical features
   a. **Signs and symptoms** include ptosis, diplopia, difficulty chewing or swallowing, respiratory difficulties, and limb weakness.
   b. **Weakness may be localized** to only a few muscle groups, especially the extraocular muscles, or may be generalized.
   c. **Weakness improves** after rest.
   d. **Sensation and reflexes** are normal.

3. Laboratory findings
   a. **Diagnosis** is **confirmed by marked improvement in muscle strength** that lasts approximately 5 to 10 minutes following a therapeutic challenge with edrophonium (an anticholinesterase inhibitor).
   b. **Posteroanterior and lateral films of the chest** (or CT scan) should be obtained to rule out a possible thymoma.
   c. **Serum acetylcholine receptor antibody titer** is elevated.
   d. **Decremental muscle response** to repetitive stimulation of motor nerves occurs.

4. Treatment

   a. Patients should **avoid aminoglycosides,** which exacerbate signs and symptoms.

   b. **Anticholinesterase drugs** (neostigmine and/or pyridostigmine) provide **symptomatic relief.**

   c. **Corticosteroids** may benefit patients who are refractory to anticholinesterase drugs.

   d. Patients who have severe signs and symptoms may benefit from **plasmapheresis.**

   e. **Thymectomy** usually leads to symptomatic relief or remission and should be considered in patients under age 60.

C. Botulism

   1. General characteristics

      a. Botulism is **caused by ingesting *Clostridium botulinum* toxin or infection with the bacterium.**

      b. The **toxin prevents the release of acetylcholine** at the neuromuscular junction.

      c. Botulism often results from **ingestion of contaminated home-canned food.**

   2. Clinical features

      a. Botulism is characterized by **sudden, fluctuating, and severe weakness** in a previously healthy person.

      b. Signs and symptoms begin **within 72 hours of ingestion of the contaminated food.**

      c. **Signs and symptoms** include diplopia, ptosis, facial weakness, and dysphagia.

      d. **Respiratory difficulty and weakness in extremities** follow.

      e. **Weakness progresses** from head to foot.

      f. Vision is **blurred,** and the **pupils** are **dilated** and unreactive.

      g. **Dry mouth, constipation, and postural hypotension** also may be present.

      h. **Sensation and reflexes** remain normal.

   3. Laboratory findings

      a. **EMG** shows normal nerve conduction velocities.

      b. **Repetitive stimulation of a motor nerve** may show a post-tetanic increase in amplitude of the evoked muscle response.

   4. Treatment

      a. Patients must be **hospitalized if ventilatory support** is required.

      b. **Polyvalent antitoxin** should be administered.

      c. **Antibiotic therapy** is not used because it may produce large quantities of toxin release as a result of bacterial death.

D. Duchenne type muscular dystrophy

   1. General characteristics

      a. Duchenne's muscular dystrophy is an **inherited disease.**

      b. Because it is an **X-linked recessive** disorder, the disease **typically affects boys.**

   2. Clinical features

      a. Affected toddlers have a **waddling, clumsy gait.**

      b. The abdomen protrudes due to **increased lumbar lordosis.**

      c. **Pseudohypertrophy of the calves** is present.

      d. Children push themselves up with their hands against their legs in order to stand.

   e. Eye movements, swallowing, and **sensation** are normal.

   f. **Mental retardation** is common.

   g. **Independent walking** is impossible by age 12.

   h. **Progressive kyphoscoliosis** and **weak respiratory muscles** are contributing factors to death, usually by the early 20s.

  3. **Laboratory findings**

   a. **Creatine kinase level** (20 to 100 times normal) is elevated before the disease is clinically evident.

   b. **Muscle biopsy** is diagnostic.

  4. Treatment

   a. **No cure** exists.

   b. **Early rehabilitation** prevents the progression of contractures, and **strength maintenance exercises** can improve the quality of life.

   c. Parents should receive **genetic counseling.**

XI. MULTIPLE SCLEROSIS (MS)

 A. General characteristics

  1. MS is an **immune-mediated destruction of myelin sheaths.**

  2. MS is **twice as common in women as in men.**

  3. MS occurs **predominantly in young adults of northern European origin.**

 B. Clinical features

  1. **Diagnosis** is based on **clinical findings.** The following **diagnostic criteria** must be met:

   a. **Two attacks** and clinical evidence of two separate lesions, or

   b. **Two attacks** with clinical evidence of one lesion and paraclinical evidence of another separate lesion.

   c. The two attacks must involve separate parts of the nervous system.

   d. If the patient has had only one attack, and the CSF is consistent with the diagnosis, the patient meets the diagnostic criteria for multiple sclerosis.

  2. **Attacks** may be variable.

  3. A young person may initially complain of being **unable to walk along an uneven surface.**

  4. **Numbness or tingling** may be present in any limb.

  5. **Spastic paresis** may develop.

  6. **Diplopia** occurs.

  7. **Tremor** may develop.

  8. **Nystagmus** occurs.

  9. **Urinary urgency or hesitancy** (sphincter disturbance) occurs.

  10. **Signs and symptoms** spontaneously **resolve,** but **relapses occur** and become more frequent with disease progression and **eventually** cause **permanent deficits.**

 C. Laboratory findings

  1. **MRI** is more helpful than CT scan in visualizing the multiple lesions.

2. **Visual and auditory evoked responses** may show prolonged latencies.

3. **CSF analysis** reveals elevated immunoglobulin G titer, which is oligoclonal in nature; this finding is highly suggestive of multiple sclerosis in the appropriate clinical setting but is not specific.

D. Treatment

1. **Progression of the disorder** cannot be prevented.

2. **Corticosteroids** may hasten recovery from relapses.

3. **Interferon therapy** may be of benefit, but it is still experimental.

8
Oncologic Diseases

I. HEAD AND NECK CARCINOMA

A. General characteristics

1. Head and neck cancer may involve oral cavity, larynx, oropharynx, or salivary glands.

2. Incidence of these cancers **increases with tobacco and alcohol consumption.**

3. These cancers are **often squamous cell tumors,** except for adenocarcinomas of the salivary glands.

B. Clinical features

1. **Signs and symptoms** include dysphagia, hoarseness, and swelling in the neck.

2. **White plaques** may be evident within the oral cavity.

3. **Neck swellings** must be **differentiated from simple lymphadenopathy** through assessment of size, firmness, and adherence to adjacent tissues.

C. Laboratory findings

1. **Biopsy** confirms the diagnosis.

2. **Computed tomography (CT) scan or magnetic resonance imaging** may be helpful in delineating the extent of the lesion.

D. Treatment

1. **Localized lesions** are treated with **surgical removal or radiotherapy.**

2. **More complex therapy** is indicated for **larger, nonresectable lesions;** this therapy is often palliative.

II. RENAL AND BLADDER CARCINOMA

A. General characteristics

1. **Renal tumors** are **usually clear cell carcinomas** (adenocarcinomas).

2. **Bladder carcinomas** are composed of **transitional cells.**

B. Clinical features

1. **Signs and symptoms of renal cancer** include flank pain, hematuria, abdominal mass that may be palpable, fatigue, anemia, and weight loss.

2. **Patients who have bladder cancer commonly have hematuria** that is usually painless; **bladder irritability and infections** may be present initially.

C. Laboratory findings

   1. **Renal tumors** may be detected with **intravenous pyelography** that may differentiate the lesion from an obstructing renal calculus.

      a. **Ultrasound** is a rapid, inexpensive test that effectively detects renal masses.

      b. **CT scan** is equally effective in detecting renal masses.

      c. **Biopsy** is required to confirm the histopathology.

   2. **Bladder tumors** are best diagnosed with **cystoscopy** and then confirmed with **biopsy.**

D. Treatment

   1. **Renal cancer** is primarily treated with **radical nephrectomy.**

   2. **Surgical resection of superficial lesions** is possible **for bladder cancer,** but more extensive lesions require cystectomy with urinary diversion.

III. PROSTATIC CARCINOMA

A. General characteristics

   1. **Incidence** of prostatic cancer **increases with age.**

   2. The carcinoma is **often widespread at the time of diagnosis** (usually involves bone).

B. Clinical features

   1. **Patients** who have prostatic cancer are **often asymptomatic.**

   2. **Signs and symptoms** include dysuria, increased urinary frequency with difficulty voiding, and back or hip pain.

   3. **Hematuria** may occur.

   4. An **elderly man with the aforementioned signs and symptoms** who does not have urethral discharge should raise the clinician's **index of suspicion for this diagnosis.**

   5. A **palpable nodule** or an **enlarged, firm, and irregularly shaped prostate** may be felt on **digital rectal examination.**

C. Laboratory findings

   1. Although **ultrasound** is effective in identifying prostate cancer, it is **not sensitive enough to be used as a screening test.**

   2. Diagnosis must be confirmed with a **biopsy.**

   3. **Serum levels of prostate-specific antigen and acid phosphatase** may be elevated; evaluation of these marker levels is useful for following the progress of patients but is **not a reliable screening tool.**

   4. **Bone marrow acid phosphatase levels** may be elevated when metastatic disease is present.

   5. **Skeletal radiographic studies** are required to detect bone metastasis.

D. Treatment

   1. **Surgery and radiotherapy** may result in a cure in early stage disease.

2. **Advanced disease** often requires **palliative treatment** that may involve **orchiectomy or** administration of **exogenous estrogen** (tumors are androgen sensitive).

IV. GASTRIC CARCINOMA

A. General characteristics

1. **Incidence** increases with low dietary intake of fruits and vegetables and high intake of starches.

2. **Incidence in Japan** is **high,** whereas **incidence in the United States** has **declined.**

3. **Gastric cancer is twice as common in men as in women.**

4. The tumor is **almost always an adenocarcinoma.**

5. The most common types of gastric carcinoma are:
  a. **Advanced carcinoma,** in which large tumors are found partly within and partly outside of the stomach.
  b. **Ulcerating carcinoma,** in which a deep, penetrating ulcer-tumor extends throughout all layers and may involve adjacent organs.
  c. **Polypoid carcinomas,** in which large, bulky, intraluminal growths metastasize late.

B. Clinical features

1. An early symptom is **vague postprandial heaviness** that becomes more frequent.

2. Patients are anorexic (**anorexia** may be pronounced for meat products).

3. **Weight loss** is the most common sign.

4. **Vomiting** may be a prominent symptom if pyloric obstruction occurs; coffee-ground vomitus is associated with a bleeding tumor.

5. **Lesions** occurring **at the cardia of the stomach** may cause dysphagia.

6. An **epigastric mass** may be palpable.

7. **Virchow's node** (left supraclavicular node) may be present if metastasis has occurred.

8. **Intra-abdominal masses** may be palpable, depending on the degree and location of metastases.

C. Laboratory findings

1. **Anemia** (iron deficiency) is present in approximately half of the patients.

2. **Stool analysis** is positive for occult blood.

3. **Carcinoembryonic antigen (CEA) level** is elevated in two thirds of patients; this result usually indicates extensive metastases.

4. **Upper gastrointestinal (GI) series** may be diagnostic, but the false-negative rate is approximately 20%.

5. **Diagnosis** is confirmed by gastroscopy with multiple biopsies.

D. Treatment

1. **Surgery** offers the only chance for cure; approximately 50% of patients have resectable lesions, and half of these patients are potentially curable (i.e., 25%).

2. **Adjuvant chemotherapy** has proved to be of little value.

V. PANCREATIC CARCINOMA

A. General characteristics

1. Pancreatic cancer is the **third leading cause of death due to cancer** (after lung and colon) **in men between ages 35 and 54.**

2. **Increased risk** occurs with smoking, fried meat and fat consumption, and African-American descent; **coffee and alcohol intake** are less strongly associated with increased incidence.

3. **Peak incidence** occurs in the fifth and sixth decades of life.

4. The tumor is **most commonly located** at the head of the gland.

5. **Tumor type** is **usually ductal adenocarcinoma** with a poorly differentiated cell pattern.

6. Pancreatic cancer is **characterized by early local extension and metastasis** to regional lymph nodes and the liver.

B. Clinical features

1. **Signs and symptoms** include weight loss, obstructive jaundice (if tumor is located at the head of the pancreas), and deep-seated abdominal pain.

2. **Pain** may radiate to the back in 25% of patients and is associated with a worse prognosis; pain may be relieved by sitting up with the spine flexed and is aggravated by recumbency.

3. **Hepatomegaly** may be present.

4. An **epigastric mass** may be palpated and is usually indicative of a nonresectable lesion.

5. A **palpable, nontender gallbladder in a patient who has jaundice** suggests neoplastic obstruction of the common bile duct (seen in 50% of patients).

6. **Jaundice** is associated with pruritus.

7. **Ascites** may be present.

C. Laboratory findings

1. **Serum bilirubin level** (average is 18 mg/dL) is much higher than that found in benign disease of the biliary tree.

2. **Aspartate aminotransferase** and **alanine aminotransferase** are usually not significantly elevated.

3. **Elevated alkaline phosphatase level** occurs when bile duct obstruction is present and/or liver metastasis has occurred.

4. Although a **serum CEA level** greater than 9 ng/dL is usually associated with extrapancreatic spread, **tumor markers** are otherwise not useful in diagnosis because of their lack of sensitivity.

5. **CT scan** reveals a pancreatic mass in nearly all patients; pancreatic and bile duct dilatation is strong evidence of the disease despite the absence of an apparent pancreatic mass.

6. **Endoscopic retrograde cholangiopancreatography** should also be performed to visualize the ductal system.

D. Treatment

1. **Surgical resection** is indicated for resectable tumors (only 20%).

2. **Jaundice and pruritus** are relieved by **choledochojejunostomy** or **placement of a biliary stent** in patients who have unresectable lesions.

3. Although **radiotherapy and chemotherapy** can provide some palliation, these therapies are not curative.

VI. COLORECTAL CARCINOMA

A. Cancer of the Colon and Rectum

1. General characteristics
   a. **Colorectal cancer** is the **second leading cause of death due to cancer** (after lung).
   b. **Incidence increases with age,** peaking in the 70s and 80s.
   c. **Carcinoma of the right colon is more common in women,** whereas **carcinoma of the rectum is more common in men.**
   d. The **majority of colorectal tumors are adenocarcinomas.**
   e. **Other conditions associated with an increased risk of colorectal cancer** include positive family history, ulcerative colitis, Crohn's disease, decreased intake of dietary fiber with an increased fat intake, and colorectal polyps.

2. Clinical features
   a. **Signs and symptoms of right colon cancer** include fatigue, weakness, and anemia.
      (1) Patients report a vague, right-sided **abdominal discomfort** that may be postprandial.
      (2) **Obstruction** is **uncommon** because of the large caliber of the right colon and the liquidity of the stool (hence, alteration in bowel habits is not a common symptom).
      (3) **Gross blood** may not be evident in the stool.
      (4) Occasionally, a **mass may be palpable** on abdominal examination.
   b. **Symptoms of left colon cancer** include increased frequency of defecation (not true watery diarrhea) alternating with constipation due to the semisolid nature of the stools and the small caliber of the left colon.
      (1) Patients may **initially** be seen with **partial or complete obstruction.**
      (2) **Stool** may be **streaked with blood/clots.**
      (3) A **mass** may be **palpable** on abdominal examination.
   c. Patients who have **rectal cancer** are **most often** seen with **hematochezia.**
      (1) **Tenesmus** may be present.
      (2) **Digital rectal examination** may reveal a flat, hard, oval, or encircling mass.
   d. **Inguinal and supraclavicular nodes** should be palpated in all bowel carcinoma patients, because enlargement of these nodes is evidence of metastasis; an enlarged node may also provide an accessible site for biopsy.
   e. **Colorectal cancer patients** may be initially seen with symptoms of obstruction, including nausea; vomiting; severe, cramping abdominal pain; and absence of flatus and bowel movements. Fever and tachycardia may also occur.

3. Laboratory findings
   a. Patients have **hypochromic, microcytic anemia.**
   b. **Urinalysis** should be performed to assess for urinary tract infections that may

result from an enterovesical fistula formed via extension and invasion of the colonic tumor.

   c. **Renal function** should be assessed via measurement of serum creatinine level.

   d. **Liver function** should be assessed because colonic cancer may metastasize to the liver (i.e., measurement of albumin, bilirubin, and transaminase levels).

   e. **Alkaline phosphatase level** should be measured to assess for early bone metastasis.

   f. **Measurement of CEA levels** is only useful in detecting recurrence of disease after curative surgical resection; it should not be used as a screening test because of its lack of sensitivity.

   g. **Barium enema** is effective in delineating the lesions (see Figure 6-7); **chest radiographic studies** should also be obtained to assess for metastasis as well as free air under the diaphragm (which suggests intestinal perforation from the colonic tumor).

   h. **Barium swallow** should **not** be **performed** because it may precipitate acute large-bowel obstruction in a patient with suspected large-bowel cancer.

   i. **Colonoscopy with biopsy** confirms the diagnosis and should be performed to assess the entire colon; colonoscopy without barium enema is becoming standard practice in most centers.

   j. **Radiographic studies** are unreliable for diagnosis of rectal cancer; rectal carcinomas are best diagnosed with a sigmoidoscopy.

   k. **CT scans** are not essential for diagnosis of colorectal cancer but may assist in assessment of disease extent.

   4. Treatment

   a. **For colonic cancer, surgical resection of the affected colon** is often performed even if metastasis is present, because removal of the lesion can prevent obstruction and hemorrhage.

   b. **For rectal cancer, surgical resection is performed** with an attempt to preserve anal sphincter function when possible; **adjuvant chemotherapy and radiotherapy** can significantly reduce the surgical resection necessary for tumor removal.

   c. **Follow-up** should include CEA determinations every 2 months and fecal occult blood testing biannually; **colonoscopy** should be performed 1 year after resection of the tumor.

B. Colonic and rectal polyps

   1. General characteristics

   a. Polyps may be **sessile or pedunculated.**

   b. Polyps may be **benign or malignant.**

   c. Most polyps are **adenomatous,** and are either tubular, tubulovillous, or villous and have neoplastic potential; sessile lesions are more likely to become malignant than are pedunculated lesions.

   d. At least **half of all polyps** occur in the **sigmoid colon or rectum.**

   e. **Other polyp types** include hyperplastic and inflammatory polyps; both are non-neoplastic.

   f. **Familial polyposis syndromes** are a rare group of diseases summarized in Table 8-1.

   2. Clinical features

   a. **Most patients who have polyps are asymptomatic; most polyps are discovered by routine sigmoidoscopy.**

   b. **Rectal bleeding** is the **most common complaint;** the bleeding is usually intermittent (rarely profuse).

Table 8-1
Familial Polyposis Syndromes

Syndrome	Symptoms/Signs	Malignant Potential
Familial adenomatous polyposis	>100 polyps in colon and rectum	Yes
Gardner's syndrome	Polyposis, desmoid tumors, osteomas, sebaceous cysts	Yes
Turcot syndrome	Polyposis, medulloblastoma/glioma	Yes
Peutz-Jeghers syndrome	Multiple hamartomatous polyps, melanotic pigmentation of skin and mucous membranes	Small

    c. Generally, patients do not report a change in **bowel habits,** unless the polyp is large.

    d. **Peristaltic cramps** may occasionally be caused by polypoid tumors.

    e. **Rectal polyps** may be felt on digital rectal examination.

  3. Laboratory findings

    a. **Anemia** is usually not present because bleeding is typically not extensive unless the polyp is malignant.

    b. **Barium enemas** may reveal a filling defect associated with the polyp(s): however, polyps less than 5 mm are generally difficult to detect.

    c. **Colonoscopy** is the most reliable means of detecting and treating small polypoid lesions.

  4. Treatment

    a. **Polyps should be removed** because they are either symptomatic (e.g., bleeding), or have malignant potential.

    b. **Colonoscopy** is an effective means of polyp removal.

VII. LUNG CARCINOMA

  A. General characteristics

    1. Lung cancer is the **most common cause of cancer deaths.**

    2. Lung cancer is **typically seen in the sixth decade of life.**

    3. **Smoking** is the **most common cause,** but **asbestos exposure** is **also associated** with this condition.

    4. **Asymptomatic individuals** have the **best chance of survival** (75% of symptomatic patients are incurable).

    5. **Mean survival time** is 9 months from time of diagnosis.

    6. The **majority of lung cancers** fall into three pathologic types: **squamous cell carcinoma, adenocarcinoma,** and **small-cell** (oat cell) **carcinoma.**

      a. Squamous cell carcinoma

        (1) Accounts for **30% of lung cancers**

        (2) **Tends to occur centrally,** near the hilum

        (3) Has **slower growth and metastatic rates** relative to other lung cancers

      b. Adenocarcinoma

        (1) Accounts for **30% of lung cancers**

        (2) May be **mucus-secreting** (acinar adenocarcinoma)

(3) May be **bronchioalveolar carcinoma** (scar-like carcinoma)

  c. Small-cell (oat cell) carcinoma:

    (1) Accounts for **25% of lung cancers**

    (2) Occurs **centrally**

    (3) Metastasizes early

    (4) Is the **most resistant to combined modality treatment**

B. Clinical features

  1. Intrathoracic signs and symptoms include cough, hemoptysis, wheezing, recurrent pneumonia, and pleuritic pain.

    a. Hoarseness occurs due to recurrent laryngeal nerve involvement.

    b. Neck or facial swelling occurs due to superior vena cava obstruction.

    c. Diaphragmatic paralysis occurs due to phrenic nerve involvement.

    d. Pancoast's syndrome, characterized by pain of the ipsilateral arm, and **Horner's syndrome** (ptosis, miosis, ipsilateral anhydrosis) are caused by a tumor of the upper lobe of the lung.

  2. Extrathoracic signs and symptoms may be due to metastasis or paraneoplastic syndromes.

    a. Metastasis commonly occurs to the liver, adrenal glands, brain, and bone.

    b. Paraneoplastic syndromes include Cushing's syndrome, hypercalcemia, syndrome of inappropriate antidiuretic hormone, neuropathies, clubbing, and hypertrophic pulmonary osteoarthropathy.

  3. Nonspecific signs and symptoms include weight loss, anorexia, weakness, and malaise.

C. Laboratory findings

  1. Microscopic analysis of sputum may reveal atypical cells; however, cell yields are often inconsistent.

  2. Some patients may have **anemia** that is consistent with chronic disease.

  3. An **atypical chest radiograph** may be the first indication of lung cancer.

    a. Cavitation and obstructive pneumonitis are more commonly seen with squamous cell carcinomas and tend to occur near the hilum.

    b. Adenocarcinoma is often seen at the periphery.

  4. Bronchoscopy with biopsy/brushings establishes the diagnosis in the majority of patients.

  5. Patients experiencing **signs and symptoms of paraneoplastic syndromes** should be evaluated.

  6. Ventilation-perfusion scan can be used to preoperatively assess pulmonary reserve.

D. Treatment

  1. Patients who have resectable lesions, that is, no distant metastases, and adequate cardiopulmonary reserve when the affected area of the lung is removed, **require surgery for cure.**

  2. Patients must be assessed for new neurologic signs and symptoms, bone pain/ tenderness, and an **elevated alkaline phosphatase level;** if these signs and symptoms are not present, routine bone and CT scans are not indicated.

  3. Nodes within the mediastinum must be assessed; if nodes are less than 1 cm in size, they are positive for metastases in less than 5% of patients.

4. **Patients who have small-cell lung carcinomas** have **better survival rates** than patients who have other carcinoma types.

5. **Radiotherapy** is used palliatively for unresectable tumors.

6. **Chemotherapy** can, in some patients, be used as an adjunct to surgery of resectable lesions.

VIII. MULTIPLE MYELOMA : *flack*.

A. General characteristics

1. Multiple myeloma is a **malignant proliferation of plasma cells derived from a single clone.**

2. **Incidence** increases with age (rare in patients < 40 years of age).

3. **Malignant myeloma** is **twice as common in African-Americans.**

B. Clinical features

1. **Bone pain** is the most common symptom (usually occurs in the back and ribs).

2. **Persistent localized pain** in a patient who has myeloma **usually** indicates a **pathologic fracture.**

3. Patients may have **signs and symptoms of spinal cord compression** secondary to vertebral fractures.

4. **Masses associated with lytic lesions of the skull** may be palpated.

5. Patients have an **increased susceptibility to bacterial infections,** that is, pneumonia and pyelonephritis; *Streptococcus pneumoniae, Staphylococcus aureus,* and *Klebsiella* species commonly cause pneumonia, whereas *Escherichia coli* is predominant in the urinary tract.

6. Patients may become **edematous secondary to renal failure,** which **commonly occurs as a result of hypercalcemia.**

7. **Hypercalcemia** may cause confusion, weakness, and lethargy.

8. **Hepatosplenomegaly** rarely occurs.

C. Laboratory findings

1. Patients have **normochromic-normocytic anemia.**

2. Urine contains **Bence Jones (M-chain) proteins.**

3. **Chest and long bone radiographic studies** reveal lytic lesions or diffuse osteopenia.

4. **Elevated levels of blood urea nitrogen and creatinine** indicate renal failure.

5. **Serum calcium level** is elevated.

6. M component is increased on **protein electrophoresis** (usually immunoglobulin G).

D. Treatment

1. **Radiotherapy** to solitary bone plasmacytomas often is curative; radiotherapy may be used palliatively as well.

2. **Chemotherapy** is also useful, for example, cyclophosphamide and prednisone.

3. **Corticosteroids, hydration,** and **natriuresis** are **indicated for hypercalcemia.**

Table 8-2
Rye Classification of Hodgkin's Lymphoma

Subtype	Proportion	Pathology	Prognosis
Lymphocyte-predominant	5–10	Predominantly normal-appearing lymphocytes	Very good
Lymphocyte-depleted	10–15	Few lymphocytes, pleomorphic cells, fibrosis	Poor
Mixed cellularity	25–40	Pleomorphic cells	Good
Nodular sclerosis	50–80	Lymphoid nodules, collagen bands	Good

4. **Uric acid nephropathy** may occur during chemotherapy (from lysis of tumor burden) and cause renal failure; nephropathy can be treated with **allopurinol.**

5. **Pneumococcal vaccines** are of little use in preventing infection.

IX. THE LYMPHOMAS

A. Hodgkin's lymphoma

1. General characteristics

   a. In the United States, Hodgkin's lymphoma has a **bimodal incidence** that **peaks at ages 15 to 35 and** also **over age 50.**

   b. The disease is **more common in men,** especially within the younger age group.

   c. **Incidence increases** in patients who have **immunodeficiencies** as well as patients who have **autoimmune diseases.**

   d. Table 8-2 lists the **four histologic subtypes.**

2. Clinical features

   a. Patients are usually first seen with a **mass or group of lymph nodes** that are firm, nonfixed, and nontender.

   b. **Adenopathy** is common in the neck and/or supraclavicular area.

   c. Approximately **50% to 60% of patients have mediastinal lymphadenopathy.**

   d. **Two percent to five percent of patients** report that the **lymph nodes are painful after alcohol ingestion.**   2-5%

   e. Patients who have **constitutional signs and symptoms** are designated as having **stage B disease,** which is associated with a **less favorable prognosis than** that for **patients who have stage A disease,** which is the designation given when there are **no constitutional signs and symptoms.**

      (1) Up to **40% of patients have low-grade fever with recurrent night sweats** (more common in older patients and those who have more advanced disease).

      (2) **Weight loss** occurs in more than **10% of patients.**

   f. **Pruritis** may be present.

   g. Generally, patients do not have **opportunistic infections** because humoral immunity is usually intact.

   h. **Hepatosplenomegaly** may be present.

3. Laboratory findings

   a. Patients who have **lymph nodes greater than 1 cm for more than 4 to 6 weeks** should undergo biopsy.

   b. Presence of **Reed-Sternberg cells** confirms the diagnosis.

   c. **Hematologic analysis** reveals normochromic-normocytic anemia, with elevated iron stores and low iron-binding capacity consistent with anemia of chronic disease.

  d. A marked leukemoid reaction is evident.

4. Treatment

  a. Staging laparotomy is often required because CT scan is not as accurate in detecting disease.

  b. Radiotherapy (localized disease—stages I and II) and chemotherapy (disseminated disease—stages III and IV) should be used with the intention of cure.

B. Non-Hodgkin's lymphoma

  1. General characteristics

    a. Peak incidence occurs in individuals between ages 20 and 40.

    b. This disease may be associated with viral infection and immunosuppression (e.g., iatrogenic or acquired immunodeficiency syndrome).

    c. The majority of subtypes are of B-cell lineage (except for the high-grade lymphoblastic subtype, which has a T-cell origin).

  2. Clinical features

    a. Persistent, painless, peripheral lymphadenopathy is common.

    b. Epitrochlear and mesenteric node involvement are more suggestive of non-Hodgkin's rather than Hodgkin's lymphoma.

    c. Patients are less likely to have constitutional signs and symptoms (compared with Hodgkin's).

    d. Site-specific signs and symptoms associated with lymphadenopathy may occur.

    e. Hepatosplenomegaly may be present.

  3. Laboratory findings

    a. Biopsy of suspicious nodes is required for diagnosis.

    b. Suggested work-up includes complete blood count, liver function tests, renal function tests, determination of alkaline phosphatase level, CT scan of the abdomen and pelvis, and bone marrow biopsy in order to determine the extent of the disease.

    c. Hypergammaglobulinemia is not present because the overproduced B cell is typically in a resting state (unlike multiple myeloma).

  4. Treatment

    a. Treatment is based on histologic subtype (low-, intermediate- or high-grade lymphoma).

    b. Radiotherapy has a limited role.

    c. Chemotherapy is the most common treatment modality.

    d. Bone marrow transplantation is of some benefit for patients who are refractory to standard chemotherapy.

X. THE LEUKEMIAS

A. General characteristics

  1. The leukemias are classified according to cell type and may be either acute or chronic, myeloid or lymphoid.

  2. Risk factors include a family history, radiation exposure, and treatment with certain chemotherapeutic agents (alkylating agents).

  3. The four main subtypes are acute lymphocytic leukemia (ALL), acute myelogenous leukemia (AML), **chronic lymphocytic leukemia (CLL)**, and **chronic my-elogenous leukemia (CML)**.

B. **Acute leukemias**

1. Acute leukemias include **acute lymphocytic leukemia** and **acute lymphoblastic leukemia.**

2. **ALL** may be **T-cell type** (20%); **null-type** (non-T, non-B cell); or, less commonly, **B-cell type.**

 a. ALL typically occurs in children.

 b. The presence of an enzyme, **terminal deoxynucleotidyl transferase,** is relatively specific for ALL.

3. **AML is characterized by larger myelogenous cells** (relative to lymphoblastic cells) **that may contain Auer bodies** (abnormal primary granules, which are a diagnostic finding).

 a. AMLs are rare in children.

 b. AMLs are not uncommon in persons receiving radiotherapy for Hodgkin's disease.

4. Clinical features

 a. **Signs and symptoms of ALL and AML** are similar.

 b. **Fatigue** is the **most common presenting symptom** and **may be associated with pallor and dyspnea on mild exertion** (symptoms of anemia).

 c. **Fever** may be present, with no obvious sign of infection.

 d. **Bone pain** occurs secondary to marrow infiltration.

 e. **Thrombocytopenia** leads to bleeding abnormalities (petechiae and easy bruising).

 f. **Oral and GI hemorrhages** begin to occur when the platelet count is below $20 \times 10^9/L$.

 g. **Decreasing levels of polymorphonuclear neutrophils (PMNs)** occurring secondary to marrow infiltration may cause frequent infections.

  (1) **Infecting organisms** may be gram-positive cocci, gram-negative organisms, and *Candida* species.

  (2) **Mucosal breakdown** leads to infection of the skin, gingiva, perirectal tissue, and lung and urinary tracts.

 h. **Hepatosplenomegaly** may be present and produce signs and symptoms of early satiety.

 i. An **anterior mediastinal mass** is usually indicative of T-cell type ALL and is not typically found in other forms of leukemia.

 j. **Soft-tissue masses of leukemic cells** can develop in any area **(chloromas).**

 k. **Generalized lymphadenopathy** may be present.

 l. **Neurologic signs and symptoms associated with leukemic meningitis** can occur (headache and nausea, followed by seizures and decreased mentation) but are **usually not present at** the time of **diagnosis.**

5. Laboratory findings

 a. **Signs typical of pancytopenia** (normochromic-normocytic anemia) **are present,** with the exception of large numbers of lymphoblasts (ALL) or myeloblasts (AML).

 b. **White blood cell count (WBC)** may be $> 50 \times 10^9/L$ or may be as low as $5 \times 10^9/L$; in either case, blastic cells predominate.

 c. **Serum lactate dehydrogenase and uric acid levels** may be increased due to increased cell turnover.

 d. **Cerebrospinal fluid** may reveal leukemic blast cells, increased protein levels, and decreased glucose levels in **leukemic meningitis.**

    e. Bone marrow biopsy confirms the diagnosis.

    f. CT scan may be useful in delineating extramedullary sites that are impinging on other structures.

6. Treatment

    a. Patients should receive **transfusion with the** appropriate **blood products; platelet count** should be maintained above $20 \times 10^9/L$.

    b. Fever must be evaluated, and the patient should be placed on **broad-spectrum antibiotics** until the cause of the fever can be found and infection is either ruled out or appropriately treated.

    c. Because **fungal infections** may also exist, a **patient who is unresponsive to antibiotics** should receive a **trial of amphotericin B; daily serum creatinine levels** should be **evaluated for** possible **nephrotoxicity** that occurs with this agent.

    d. The use of **granulocyte transfusions** remains **controversial.**

    e. Fifty percent of children who have ALL are cured with chemotherapy.

    f. Because **treatment** often leads to increased serum urate levels, **allopurinol** (which decreases formation of uric acid) and **diuretics** may be necessary to **prevent** the **formation of urate renal calculi.**

    g. Only 10% to 30% of patients who have AML survive for more than 5 years disease-free despite treatment with chemotherapy.

    h. Acute promyelocytic leukemia (a subtype of AML) is **often associated with disseminated intravascular coagulopathy;** patients who have this subtype often require **prophylactic heparin therapy** during chemotherapy.

C. Chronic lymphocytic leukemia

1. General characteristics

    a. CLL is characterized by accumulation of mature-appearing lymphocytes in the peripheral blood and **infiltration** of these lymphocytes **into the marrow, spleen, and lymph nodes.**

    b. This disease **usually occurs in individuals over age 50.**

    c. The disease is **more common in men** and is the **most common form of chronic leukemia in the United States.**

    d. CLL is **most often caused by a clonal expansion of B cells.**

2. Clinical features

    a. CLL may be discovered **incidentally.**

    b. Patients may **initially** be seen with **signs and symptoms of anemia** such as fatigue, pallor, and dyspnea on exertion.

    c. Lymphadenopathy may be present.

    d. Intercurrent infection (decreased levels of mature PMNs) may be present.

    e. Patients who have **advanced disease** may have **easy bruising** and **gingival bleeding** (thrombocytopenia).

    f. Hepatosplenomegaly may be noted.

3. Laboratory findings

    a. Normochromic-normocytic anemia is present.

    b. WBC ranges between 15 and 200 $\times 10^9/L$, with a predominance of mature-appearing lymphocytes.

    c. Lymph node biopsy may be necessary to **distinguish a normal reactive lymphocytosis from CLL.**

    d. An **M spike** demonstrated **on protein electrophoresis** similar to that seen in multiple myeloma may be present.

4. Treatment
    a. Cure is **usually not achieved** despite chemotherapy.
    b. The **goal** of treatment **is palliative.**
    c. Because **progression of the disease** is **typically slow,** patients do not receive therapy unless **cytopenia** (e.g., significant anemia or thrombocytopenia) or **marked systemic symptoms** exist.
    d. Patients may live **10 to 15 years after diagnosis** of the disease.

D. Chronic myelogenous leukemia

  1. General characteristics
    a. **CML** is characterized by **increased numbers of granulocytes** (neutrophils).
    b. The disease **generally** runs a **mild course** (chronic phase) until the development of the blastic phase.
    c. CML **can occur at any age,** but **peak incidence** occurs **between the third and fourth decades of life.**

  2. Clinical features
    a. Patients may initially be seen with **upper left quadrant abdominal discomfort** associated with splenomegaly (often palpable on physical examination).
    b. Patients have **signs and symptoms of anemia,** such as pallor, fatigue, and dyspnea on exertion.
    c. **Lymphadenopathy** is typically not present during the chronic phase of the disease.
    d. **Weight loss and fever** may be present.
    e. **Meningeal leukemia** is rare.
    f. **Blastic phase** is associated with marked anemia, thrombocytopenia (easy bruising), and predominance of blasts.

  3. Laboratory findings
    a. **Normochromic-normocytic anemia** is present.
    b. **Leukocytosis** is prominent; **myelocytes and metamyelocytes** are present (unlike a physiologic leukemoid reaction).
    c. **Basophilia** is often prominent.
    d. **Serum vitamin B_{12} levels** and **vitamin B_{12}–binding capacity** are elevated; this reflects an **increase in transcobalamin I** that is produced by the leukemic cells.
    e. **Leukocyte alkaline phosphatase level** is **decreased;** this feature **distinguishes CML from other myeloproliferative disorders.**
    f. **Hyperuricemia** occurs due to increased cell turnover.
    g. **Philadelphia chromosome** is present in more than 95% of CML patients.
    h. **Bone marrow biopsy** reveals a myeloid infiltrate.

  4. Treatment
    a. **True remission** does not occur with treatment; however, the **tumor cell mass** can be significantly reduced to enable maturation of normal cell lines.
    b. **Busulfan** is the most commonly used chemotherapeutic agent for treatment of the chronic phase of the disease.
    c. During **blastic crisis, treatment with vincristine and prednisone** may be helpful, but patients often succumb to infections or bleeding (average survival after diagnosis is 4 years).

9

Hematologic Diseases

I. ANEMIAS

A. General characteristics

1. Anemias occur because of lack of red blood cell formation, increased red blood cell destruction, blood loss, or an association with a primary disease (Table 9-1).

2. Anemias are best evaluated in terms of **red blood cell indices.** Anemia types are characterized by a mean corpuscular volume (MCV) as follows: hypochromic-microcytic anemia (MCV < 80); normochromic-normocytic anemia (MCV 80–100); and macrocytic anemia (MCV > 100) (Table 9-2).

B. Clinical features

1. Anemia types vary in **rapidity of onset.**

2. **Rapid blood loss** or **hemolysis** leads to tachycardia, postural hypotension, faintness, and peripheral vascular constriction (cold, pale extremities).

3. If anemia occurs gradually, the **plasma volume** expands to accommodate the blood loss or hemolysis, in which case the patient may notice only exertional dyspnea.

4. **Pronounced anemia** may cause pallor of skin and mucous membranes; jaundice; chelosis (fissuring of the angles of the mouth); beefy red, smooth tongue; and koilonychia (spoon-shaped nails).

5. **Additional signs** include systolic murmurs and bounding pulses with widened pulse pressures.

C. Hypochromic-microcytic anemias

1. General characteristics

   a. These anemias are caused by an **abnormality in heme or globin synthesis** (Figure 9-1).

   b. The **most common cause** is **iron deficiency** secondary to chronic blood loss or low dietary intake (seen mainly in children or pregnant women).

   c. **Other causes** include anemia of chronic disease, which results in poor iron utilization; sideroblastic anemia, which leads to a block in heme synthesis; hemoglobinopathies such as sickle-cell disease or defective globin synthesis as seen in the thalassemias.

2. **Iron deficiency**

   a. General characteristics

      (1) Iron deficiency is most often **secondary to chronic bleeding of the gastrointestinal (GI) tract.**

Table 9-1
Normal Blood Measurements

Important Values	Male	Female
Hemoglobin	13.7–17.5 g/dL	11.5–15.5 mg/dL
Red blood cells	4.5–6.5 × 10^{12}/L	3.9–5.6 × 10^{12}/L
Hematocrit	40%–52%	35%–47%

(2) It may also be **secondary to partial gastrectomy** (which impairs iron absorption) or malabsorption syndromes.

(3) Patients have the aforementioned clinical features in addition to **pica** (cravings for ice, clay, or starch).

b. Laboratory findings

(1) **Red blood cell smear** reveals hypochromic-microcytic cells.

(2) **Increased platelet count** may be noted if chronic bleeding is the cause (Table 9-3).

(3) **Serum iron level** is decreased, and total iron binding capacity (TIBC) is elevated; that is, transferrin saturation is less than 15%, ferritin is decreased, and free erythrocyte protoporphyrin (a precursor of heme that requires iron for formation) is increased.

c. Treatment

(1) An **underlying cause** should always be investigated; menstruation should never be assumed to cause a woman's iron deficiency.

(2) **Iron salts** (e.g., ferrous sulfate), 325 mg three times a day, are indicated.

(3) **Adequate therapy** results in an increase of 1 g of hemoglobin (Hgb) in 2 weeks; therefore, **noncompliance** or **continued bleeding** may be the cause if the patient is unresponsive to therapy.

3. Anemia of chronic disease

a. General characteristics

(1) Anemia of chronic disease may be **normochromic-normocytic** or **hypochromic-microcytic.**

(2) **Development** of this anemia type occurs 1 to 2 months after onset of chronic disease.

(3) **Chronic disease** leads to decreased availability of iron for erythropoiesis.

b. Laboratory findings

(1) **Serum iron** is decreased.

(2) Unlike iron deficiency, **serum ferritin** level is elevated, and TIBC is decreased.

Table 9-2
Normal Red Cell Indices

Red Blood Cell Indices	Values
Mean corpuscular Hgb	27–34 pg
Mean corpuscular volume (MCV)	80–100 fL
Mean corpuscular Hgb concentration	30–35 g/dL

Hgb = hemoglobin.

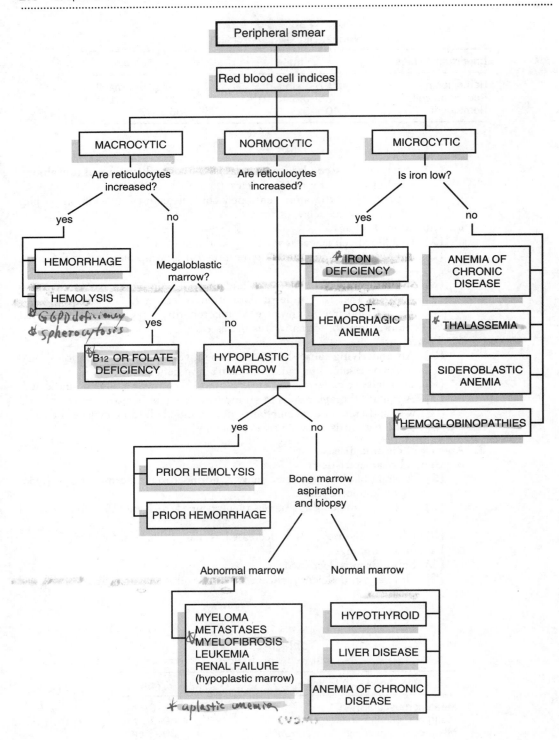

Figure 9-1. Diagnostic approach to anemias.

Table 9-3

Normal Concentration of Blood Components

Other Parameters	Values
Platelets	150–440 × 10^9/L
Reticulocyte count	0.5–2.0% (of normal RBCs)
Segmented neutrophils	2.5–7.5 × 10^9/L (50–70%)
Bands	0.1–0.6 × 10^9/L (2–6%)
Lymphocytes	1.0–5.0 × 10^9/L (20–45%)
Monocytes	0.1–1.0 × 10^9/L (2–9%)
Eosinophils	0.0–0.4 × 10^9/L (0–4%)
Basophils	0.0–0.2 × 10^9/L (0–2%)

RBC = red blood cells.

  c. Treatment
    (1) Usually, the anemia is mild and requires no treatment.
    (2) Anemia resolves when the underlying disease is treated.

4. Sideroblastic anemia
  a. General characteristics
    (1) Sideroblastic anemia is caused by a **defect in heme synthesis** that leads to iron overload secondary to ineffective erythropoiesis.
    (2) This type of anemia is **most often secondary to agents such as alcohol or lead.**
  b. Laboratory findings
    (1) **Peripheral smear** reveals hypochromic-microcytic red blood cells and rings within the red blood cells (ringed sideroblasts).
    (2) **Serum iron and ferritin levels** are elevated.
  c. Treatment
    (1) The **offending agents** should be **discontinued.**
    (2) **Transfusions** may be necessary if the degree of anemia is significant.

5. Sickle-cell disease
  a. General characteristics
    (1) Sickle-cell disease is **caused by a mutated form of the beta-globin chain (Hgb S),** which is insoluble under deoxygenated conditions and **causes sickle-shaped red blood cells.**
    (2) The disease is **most common in blacks.**
    (3) Individuals may be **homozygous** for the defective gene and have **severe** anemia, or they may be **heterozygous** and have **mild** anemia.
  b. Clinical features
    (1) Signs and symptoms begin in infancy when fetal hemoglobin (Hgb F) levels fall.
    (2) **Signs** include painful crises; swelling of extremities and spleen; and bony, pulmonary, and cerebral infarctions.
    (3) **Microvascular occlusion** from abnormally shaped red blood cells (RBCs) leads to infarction of virtually any organ.
    (4) **Chronic hemolysis** leads to increased incidence of cholelithiasis with bilirubin stones.
    (5) **Splenic infarction** leads to increased susceptibility to encapsulated organisms (e.g., *Streptococcus pneumoniae*).

c. Laboratory findings

   (1) **Peripheral smear** reveals sickle-shaped cells, elevated reticulocyte count (>20%), and nucleated RBCs.

   (2) **Serum analysis** reveals elevated bilirubin level (mainly conjugated) and low free haptoglobin (hemoglobin-binding protein) level.

   (3) **Hemoglobin electrophoresis** reveals the abnormal Hgb S.

d. Treatment

   (1) Treatment is largely **symptomatic.**

   (2) **Painful crises** are managed with oxygen therapy, fluids, correction of acidosis, and analgesics.

   (3) Because sickle-cell crisis itself does not cause fever, **infection** must be suspected in a patient who has fever, because the infection can precipitate a crisis.

   (4) **Pneumococcal vaccine** must be administered to all patients.

   (5) Although **acute crises** are not alleviated by transfusions, **chronic exchange transfusions** may decrease iron overload, reduce anemia, and lessen the degree of sickling.

6. Thalassemias

a. General characteristics

   (1) Two types of thalassemias exist: *α*-thalassemia and *β*-thalassemia; both are congenital.

   (2) Each type may occur **homozygously** (more severe disease) or **heterozygously** (minor disease).

   (3) The **minor forms** are typically benign and require no therapy.

b. Beta-thalassemia major

   (1) General characteristics

   (a) Virtually all patients **die before the third decade of life.**

   (b) A **defect in the beta subunit of hemoglobin** → precipitation of alpha chains → hemolytic red blood cell destruction → ineffective erythropoiesis → hyperplastic bone marrow, liver, and spleen.

   (c) This type of thalassemia is **most common in individuals of Mediterranean descent.**

   (2) Clinical features

   (a) **Signs and symptoms** do not occur until **age 4 to 6 months** when the **switch from fetal to adult hemoglobin** occurs.

   (b) Patients have **signs and symptoms of severe anemia.**

   (c) Patients have **marked wasting** and a **malnourished** appearance.

   (d) **Chipmunk facies** are present.

   (e) **Marked hepatosplenomegaly** occurs.

   (f) **Growth retardation** and **fractures** occur secondary to **excessive bone marrow expansion.**

   (3) Laboratory findings

   (a) **Hemoglobin analysis** reveals persistence of Hgb F.

   (b) **Peripheral smear** reveals hypochromic-microcytic anemia, many nucleated red blood cells, and anisocytosis.

   (c) Hgb level is usually between 3 and 6 mg/dl in the untreated state.

   (4) Treatment

   (a) Treatment of major disease involves **transfusion therapy.**

   (b) **Desferrioxamine** may be required to prevent iron overload from repeated transfusions.

   (c) **Splenectomy** may be required to decrease red blood cell destruction.

c. Alpha-thalassemia

(1) Two clinically significant forms of the disease exist: Hgb H disease and Bart's Hgb (gamma$_4$ chains).

(2) **Bart's Hgb** leads to hydrops fetalis; in utero, the total absence of alpha chains leads to 100% gamma Hgb, which binds oxygen tightly and therefore deprives tissues of oxygen.

(3) **Hgb H disease** is characterized by beta$_4$ chains that tend to precipitate within the red blood cells (Heinz bodies), which leads to hemolytic anemia.

(a) **Signs and symptoms** are similar to β-thalassemia, but they are often less severe.

(b) **Treatment** is similar to that for β-thalassemia.

D. **Normochromic-normocytic anemias**

1. **General characteristics**

a. These disorders can be classified as anemias in which bone marrow production is impaired and anemias in which red blood cell production is normal.

b. **Anemias in which bone marrow production is impaired** include aplastic anemia, myelophthisic syndromes, and red blood cell aplasia.

c. Normochromic-normocytic anemias may also occur as a **result of anemia of chronic disease** (see hypochromic-microcytic anemias, I C).

d. **Anemias in which erythropoietic response is normal** include anemia of hemorrhage and hemolytic anemias (may be macrocytic due to the predominance of reticulocytes; see macrocytic anemias, I E).

2. **Aplastic anemia**

a. **General characteristics**

(1) Aplastic anemia produces a **peripheral pancytopenia,** but bone marrow architecture is unaffected.

(2) This form of anemia may be **inherited** (Fanconi's anemia), **secondary to viral infection** [hepatitis, Epstein-Barr virus (EBV)], or **drug-induced** (cytosine arabinoside, chloramphenicol, phenylbutazone).

b. **Clinical features**

(1) **Severity of signs and symptoms** reflects the progression of the disease.

(2) **Neutropenia** predisposes patients to infection.

(3) Patients with **thrombocytopenia** may have petechiae and purpura.

c. **Laboratory findings**

(1) **Corrected reticulocyte count** is $< 1\%$, **platelet count** is $< 20.0 \times 10^9/$L, and **polymorphonuclear neutrophil (PMN) count** $< 0.5 \times 10^9/$L.

(2) **Bone marrow aspiration** reveals a hypoplastic marrow without evidence of infiltration.

d. **Treatment**

(1) **Blood transfusions** should be given as required.

(2) **Bone marrow transplantation** may also be effective if the appropriate donor is found.

3. **Myelophthisic syndromes (myelofibrosis)**

a. **General characteristics**

(1) Myelophthisic syndromes are **caused by invasion of the bone marrow by infection** (TB); **tumor** (breast, lung, prostate, thyroid, leukemia, lymphoma, myeloma); or **fibrosis.**

(2) **Invasion** leads to anemia, thrombocytopenia, and leukocytosis. w.c.↑

b. **Clinical features**

(1) Patients experience an insidious onset of **weight loss, weakness, and pallor.**

(2) Splenomegaly $\rightarrow$ platelet trapping $\rightarrow$ bleeding and petechiae.

    c. Laboratory findings

       (1) **Peripheral smear** reveals normochromic-normocytic cells, normoblasts, teardrop cells, inappropriately decreased reticulocyte count, and elevated white blood cell (WBC) count with a "shift to the left" (immature WBCs).

       (2) **Bone marrow aspiration** yields a dry tap due to the infiltration by abnormal tissue.

       (3) **Bone marrow biopsy** must therefore be performed to reveal the abnormal marrow architecture.

    d. Treatment

       (1) The **primary pathologic process** must be treated.

       (2) **Blood transfusions** may be necessary.

  4. **Red blood cell aplasia**

    a. Red blood cell aplasia is characterized by **anemia with no evidence of reticulocytosis.**

    b. **Platelet and WBC counts** are normal; **bone marrow** is also normal, except for the absence of erythroid precursors.

    c. Red blood cell aplasia is associated with **immunologic deficiency states** (including thymoma).

    d. It may also be **drug-induced** (chlorpropamide, gold, isoniazid).

    e. **Clinical features** are similar to those of anemia.

    f. **Treatment** involves red blood cell transfusions.

E. Macrocytic anemias

  1. Macrocytic anemias include **anemias caused by reticulocytosis,** that is, acute hemorrhage and hemolytic anemias, as well as the **megaloblastic anemias.**

  2. **Acute hemorrhage**

    (a) An acute hemorrhage is characterized by a **clinically apparent site of bleeding** (trauma, GI tract).

    (b) Patients develop **compensatory reticulocytosis.**

    (c) Patients have **signs and symptoms of acute blood loss,** that is, tachycardia, hypotension, sweating, pallor, and cold and clammy extremities.

    (d) **Rapid replacement of blood products** may be required if hemorrhage is significant.

  3. Hemolytic anemias

    a. **Intravascular hemolytic anemia**

       (1) General characteristics

          (a) This type of anemia is **caused by acute transfusion reactions** (antibody-mediated), **prosthetic heart valve dysfunction, cold agglutinin disease,** or **clostridial infection.**

          (b) **RBC destruction** → free hemoglobin binding to haptoglobin, hemopexin, and/or albumin (methemoglobin) → clearance by the liver; the **binding capacity of haptoglobin/albumin** is often exceeded, which leads to **hemoglobinuria.**

          (c) **Chronic hemolysis** leads to renal tubular cells filled with hemosiderin that is sloughed into urine, which leads to **iron deficiency.**

       (2) Clinical features

          (a) Patients have **signs and symptoms of anemia.**

          (b) Restlessness, anxiety, flushing, fever and chills, headache, chest or lumbar pain, tachypnea, and nausea may indicate an **acute transfusion reaction.**

          (c) The **transfusion reaction** may progress to shock, renal failure, and disseminated intravascular coagulation (DIC).

(3) Laboratory findings

    (a) Serum **free haptoglobin** and **hemopexin levels** are decreased.

    (b) **Plasma** and **urine hemoglobin levels** are elevated; **lactate dehydrogenase (LDH) level** is elevated; and **total and indirect (unconjugated) bilirubin levels** are elevated.

    (c) **Peripheral smear** reveals macrocytic anemia with reticulocytosis, nucleated red blood cells, and cell fragments.

    (d) **Coombs' test** (which detects the presence of RBC antibodies) is **positive** if the anemia is antibody-mediated; the test is **negative** if the anemia is secondary to shearing from prosthetic valve dysfunction.

(4) Treatment

    (a) Immediate therapy with an **osmotic diuretic** to decrease the risk of renal damage is necessary.

    (b) **Patients** should be **hospitalized** for appropriate management of shock and DIC.

b. **Extravascular hemolysis**

(1) General characteristics

    (a) This disease is **caused by** the **abnormally early removal of RBCs** by the spleen and liver.

    (b) Because only a small amount of Hgb is released into the blood vessels to bind with other proteins, **iron deficiency** is **less likely** to occur.

    (c) Extravascular hemolysis is **often associated with antibodies to the Rhesus factor.**

(2) Clinical features

    (a) Signs and symptoms usually include **malaise and fever.**

    (b) **Shock and renal failure** almost never occur.

    (c) Patients have **mild-to-moderate splenomegaly.**

(3) Laboratory findings

    (a) **Haptoglobin level** is only slightly decreased (in contrast to intravascular hemolysis), and **hemoglobinemia** or **hemoglobinuria** does not occur.

    (b) **Indirect (unconjugated) bilirubin level** is elevated if the hemolysis is brisk.

    (c) **Serum LDH level** is elevated.

    (d) **Reticulocytosis** is present.

(4) **Treatment** is conservative and usually does not include transfusion.

c. Intracorpuscular abnormalities

(1) Hereditary spherocytosis

    (a) General characteristics

        (i) Hereditary spherocytosis is the **most common RBC membrane defect.**

        (ii) This disease is **most common in Europeans;** the **severe form** is **autosomal dominant** (therefore, the disease is often linked to a prominent family history).

        (iii) **Increased splenic destruction of RBCs** occurs secondary to altered sodium cell membrane permeability and RBC shape; because RBCs are destroyed by the spleen, this disease is considered to be a form of extravascular hemolysis.

        (iv) Cells have a decreased surface-to-volume ratio.

    (b) Clinical features

        (i) Patients who have the severe form are **first seen in childhood with jaundice** and **fatigue.**

        (ii) **Splenomegaly** is present.

       (iii) Patients have a **high incidence of gallstones** secondary to increased bilirubin turnover.

       (iv) Patients can develop **aplastic crisis.**

   (c) Laboratory findings

       (i) **Peripheral smear** reveals reticulocytosis and spherocytes.

       (ii) **Serum analysis** indicates indirect hyperbilirubinemia.

       (iii) During the **osmotic fragility test,** spherocytes lyse at lower concentrations of sodium chloride than do normal RBCs.

   (d) Treatment

       (i) **Transfusions** are necessary during aplastic crisis.

       (ii) **Splenectomy** decreases hemolysis and therefore restores the RBC life span to nearly normal; **pneumococcal vaccine** is required due to increased susceptibility in splenectomized patients.

(2) Glucose-6-phosphate dehydrogenase (G6PD) deficiency

   (a) **General characteristics**

       (i) G6PD is the **most common RBC enzyme defect.**

       (ii) **Incidence** is higher in black individuals and persons of Mediterranean descent.

       male **(iii)** This **X-linked disorder** causes a buildup of intracellular methemoglobin, which precipitates in the RBC→these precipitates are cleared in the spleen via microcytosis of red blood cell membrane→microspherocytes.

       (iv) **Lack of this enzyme** also leads to a buildup of intracellular oxidants that causes cell lysis (intravascular hemolysis).

       (v) **Exacerbations** are brought on by infection; certain drugs (antimalarials, sulfonamides); and fava beans.

   (b) **Clinical features**

       (i) Patients have **splenomegaly** and an increased incidence of **cholelithiasis.**

       (ii) **Clinical features of intravascular hemolysis** may occur.

   (c) Laboratory findings

       (i) **Peripheral smear** reveals microspherocytes (not normal-sized as seen in hereditary spherocytosis), reticulocytosis, and Heinz bodies.

       (ii) **Serum analysis** reveals decreased haptoglobin levels, hemoglobinemia, and indirect bilirubinemia.

       (iii) **Decreased intracellular G6PD activity** is evident.

   (d) Treatment

       (i) Therapy is **symptomatic; fluids and transfusions** are given as required.

       (ii) Patients should **avoid oxidants.**

4. Megaloblastic anemias

   a. General characteristics

       (1) These anemias are **commonly caused by B_{12} and/or folate deficiency.**

       (2) Impaired deoxyribonucleic acid synthesis→pancytopenia.

       (3) Destruction of developing cells by hemolysis leads to ineffective erythropoiesis.

       (4) Folate deficiency may be secondary to poor diet (commonly seen in alcoholics), malabsorption syndromes, or certain drugs (phenytoin); **body stores of folate** last 2 to 4 months; therefore, folate deficiency occurs before B_{12} deficiency.

(5) B_{12} **deficiency** is **often associated with** pernicious anemia [indicated by the presence of anti–intrinsic factor (IF) antibodies], **previous gastrectomy,** or small bowel disease (Crohn's disease, tropical sprue); B_{12} **deficiency causes** subacute combined degeneration of the spinal cord.

b. Clinical features

(1) B_{12} **and folate deficiencies** lead to sore tongue, diarrhea, and anorexia.

(2) Lack of B_{12} leads to peripheral nerve and spinal neuron demyelination, which causes paresthesias, weakness, diminished position, and vibration sense and ataxia; effects on the cerebrum may lead to dementia.

(3) Signs and symptoms of anemia are seen in both deficiencies.

c. Laboratory findings

(1) Serum B_{12} **or folate levels** are decreased, and **LDH level** is elevated; **hyperbilirubinemia** is present.

(2) Peripheral smear reveals macrocytic anemia with decreased reticulocyte response, leukopenia, hypersegmented PMNs, and large platelets with thrombocytopenia.

(3) Schilling test result is positive in pernicious anemia (B_{12} deficiency).

    (a) In this test, the patient is given a dose of nonlabeled vitamin B_{12}, followed by an oral dose of radiolabeled vitamin B_{12}; a 48-hour urine sample is then collected.

    (b) If less than 5% labeled vitamin B_{12} is found in the urine, **malabsorption of vitamin B_{12}** is suggested.

    (c) The defect is corrected with oral administration of intrinsic factor if the patient has pernicious anemia.

    (d) If no correction occurs with IF treatment, **malabsorption within the small bowel** is likely.

(4) Bone marrow changes (increased marrow iron and hyperplasia, with increased mitotic figures) are evident, but their presence is not necessary for diagnosis.

d. Treatment

(1) Administration of the appropriate vitamin leads to **bone marrow changes** within 24 to 48 hours, **reticulocytosis** within 3 to 4 days, **normalization of leukopenia and thrombocytopenia** within 10 days, **decreased bilirubin and LDH levels** within 1 to 3 weeks, **correction of anemia** within 1 to 2 months, and **correction of neurologic deficits** (in B_{12} deficiency) within 6 to 12 months if neuronal death has not occurred.

(2) In pernicious anemia, **administration of vitamin B_{12}** must be intramuscular, because oral absorption is defective.

(3) The clinician must not assume that a megaloblastic anemia is due to folate deficiency without checking for B_{12} deficiency; **folate therapy** will not correct the neuronal damage caused by a lack of vitamin B_{12}.

II. HEMATOCRIT DISORDERS

A. General characteristics

1. These disorders result from **increased red blood cell mass,** that is, elevated hematocrit.

2. Elevated hematocrit may be secondary to stress (relative) erythrocytosis or absolute erythrocytosis.

B. Stress erythrocytosis

1. General characteristics

a. Stress erythrocytosis **typically affects obese, hypertensive, tense men.**

    b. This condition is **not a true erythrocytosis** because red blood cell mass is normal (plasma volume is contracted).

  2. Clinical features

    a. **Signs and symptoms** include dizziness, headache, epistaxis, and a characteristic "ruddy" cyanosis.

    b. **Splenomegaly** is absent (unlike polycythemia vera).

  3. Laboratory findings

    a. **Hematocrit** is between 55% and 60%.

    b. **Platelets, leukocytes,** and **red blood cell mass** are normal.

  4. **Treatment** is unnecessary because the condition is generally benign.

C. Absolute erythrocytosis

  1. General characteristics

    a. This condition is characterized by a **definite increase in red blood cell mass.**

    b. **Causes** include chronic hypoxia (lung disease, heart failure); erythropoietin-secreting tumors (renal tumors); and polycythemia vera (which is caused by autonomous bone marrow).

  2. Polycythemia vera

    a. Clinical features

      (1) This condition causes **hyperviscosity,** which leads to decreased cerebral blood flow; patients have tinnitus, light-headedness, and (rarely) stroke.

      (2) **Congestive heart failure** may be present.

      (3) **Thrombosis** may be present.

    b. Laboratory findings

      (1) **Red blood cell mass** is elevated, and **arterial oxygen saturation** is more than 92% (i.e., the erythrocytosis is not secondary to hypoxia); **splenomegaly** is present.

      (2) **Alkaline phosphatase** and **serum vitamin B$_{12}$ levels** are elevated; **leukocytosis and thrombocytosis** are also present.

      (3) **Erythropoietin** is nearly absent.

    c. Treatment

      (1) **Repeated phlebotomies** are necessary to bring the hematocrit to less than 50%.

      (2) **Chemotherapy** (hydroxyurea) may be necessary for resistant cases.

III. LEUKOCYTE DISORDERS

A. Lymphopenia

  1. General characteristics

    a. Lymphopenia may be **secondary to another condition** (acute infection, elevated cortisol level), but **antibody production** is not affected.

    b. Lymphopenia that causes immunodeficiency is **most likely secondary to human immunodeficiency virus infection or a congenital disease** (if signs and symptoms appear in infancy).

    c. Lymphopenia is **usually caused by lack of T cells** (thymic hypoplasia).

    d. **B cells** may also be deficient (Bruton's agammaglobulinemia).

  2. Clinical features

    a. **T-cell deficiency** may be associated with rashes, eczema, and mucocutaneous candidiasis.

b. In **acquired immunodeficiency syndrome,** opportunistic viral, fungal, and protozoal infections predominate (*Pneumocystis carinii* pneumonia, *Mycobacterium avium-intracellulare* pneumonia or disseminated disease, hepatitis, cytomegalovirus, herpes).

c. **B-cell deficiency** is associated with repeated infections by encapsulated organisms (*Streptococcus pneumoniae*).

3. Laboratory findings
   a. **Lymphocyte count** $<1.5 \times 10^9/L$ (or $<10\%$).
   b. **Bone marrow** is usually normocellular (5% to 20% of bone marrow cells are lymphocytes).
   c. **T-cell count** is decreased.
   d. **Quantitation of immunoglobulins** is useful in detecting B-lymphocyte deficiencies.

4. Treatment
   a. **Thymic transplantation for thymic hypoplasia** has some benefit.
   b. Therapy is **supportive** with appropriate **antibiotics.**

B. Lymphocytosis
   1. General characteristics
      a. Lymphocytosis may be **caused by infection,** that is, a reactive lymphocytosis caused by EBV, hepatitis, or cytomegalovirus.
      b. Lymphocytosis can also be **caused by leukemias and lymphomas.**

   2. Clinical features
      a. **Malaise, fever, exanthem, and pharyngitis** are common.
      b. If the cause is reactive, **duration** is less than 6 weeks.
      c. **Lymphadenopathy,** usually cervical, may be present.

   3. Laboratory findings
      a. **Peripheral smear that reveals anisocytotic, atypical lymphocytes** indicates reactive process; **morphologic monotony** suggests neoplastic disease.
      b. **Serologic testing for viral causes** can help differentiate between reactive and neoplastic disease.
      c. **T- and B-cell immunocytochemistry** may identify malignant markers present on lymphocytes.

   4. Treatment
      a. **For reactive lymphocytosis,** treatment is supportive, because the disease resolves spontaneously.
      b. **Chemotherapy for neoplasms** may be required (see Chapter 8, "Oncologic Diseases").

C. Neutrophilia
   1. General characteristics
      a. Neutrophilia is **usually secondary to infection** (neutrophil count is usually $> 20 \times 10^9/L$).
      b. Neutrophilia **may also be present in inflammatory diseases.**
      c. The **most common malignancy** associated with neutrophilia is **chronic myelogenous leukemia** (CML).
      d. Neutrophilia can also be **drug-induced** (e.g., heparin, digitalis).

   2. Clinical features
      a. If the **cause** is **infectious,** patients have **signs and symptoms of infection,** that is, fever, localized pain, swelling, and purulent exudates.
      b. **Splenomegaly** is present in CML.

3. Laboratory findings
   a. **WBC count** is elevated in CML.
   b. **Serum alkaline phosphatase level** is decreased in CML.
   c. **Bone marrow aspiration** is indicated if WBC $> 20 \times 10^9$/L or increased intracellular granules are noted.
      (1) **Bone marrow cellularity** is normal if neutrophilia is secondary to acute infection.
      (2) The presence of a **significant number** of **blasts** suggests CML.
   d. **Karyotyping** should be performed to look for the **Philadelphia chromosome** (marker for CML).
   e. **Peripheral WBC count** $> 100 \times 10^9$/L occurs with CML, as does **thrombocytosis.**

4. Treatment
   a. **Infection** is treated with **appropriate antibiotic therapy.**
   b. **CML** should be **treated** appropriately (see Chapter 8, "Oncologic Diseases").

D. Neutropenia

1. **General characteristics**
   a. Neutropenia is **most commonly secondary to exogenous factors such as infections** (hepatitis, influenza) **or certain drugs** (phenothiazines, antithyroid drugs, chemotherapeutic agents).
   b. Neutropenia is **often a feature of collagen vascular diseases** (e.g., systemic lupus erythematosus).
   c. Neutropenia is also a **feature of leukemias, lymphomas,** or **myelofibrosis.**

2. **Clinical features**
   a. Neutropenia is apparent in **agranulocytosis** (neutrophil count $< 0.5 \times 10^9$/L).
   b. **Signs and symptoms** include high fever, necrotic pharyngitis, regional lymphadenopathy, and proctitis.
   c. **Cellulitis, pneumonia,** and **urinary tract infections** ensue.
   d. **Mortality** is high without treatment.

3. Laboratory findings
   a. **Peripheral neutrophil count** is $< 1.5 \times 10^9$/L.
   b. **Hypocellular marrow** revealed after bone marrow aspiration and biopsy suggests **chemical-induced toxicity;** evidence of **neoplastic disease or myelofibrosis** may be apparent.
   c. **Presence of antinuclear antibodies** indicates that **collagen vascular diseases** may be present.

4. Treatment
   a. Patients should **discontinue** possible **toxic agents.**
   b. **Infection** is treated with broad-spectrum antibiotics (ampicillin and gentamicin are common choices).
   c. **Granulocyte transfusions** are usually of little benefit.

E. Dysfunctional neutrophils

1. **General characteristics**
   a. Although these **conditions are rare,** they have **serious clinical effects.**
   b. These conditions include **chronic granulomatous disease (CGD)** and **myeloperoxidase deficiency.**
   c. CGD is **X-linked recessive;** in this disease, **PMNs lack superoxide,** which causes increased susceptibility to *Staphylococcus,* gram-negative organisms, and fungi.

   d. **Myeloperoxidase deficiency** is autosomal recessive; in this disease, patients have an **increased susceptibility to catalase-positive organisms** (e.g., *Staphylococcus aureus*).

2. **Clinical features**
   a. Clinical features are **secondary to infection.**
   b. Patients may have **fever, regional lymphadenopathy,** and **eczematoid skin eruptions.**

3. **Laboratory findings**
   a. **Granulocytosis** indicates infection.
   b. **Bone marrow aspiration** reveals granulomas in CGD and hyperplasia in infection.
   c. In the **nitroblue tetrazolium dye test,** normal PMNs digest the dye, which causes blue granule formation; **digestion and granule formation** do not occur in CGD.
   d. **Myeloperoxidase stain** is not apparent in myeloperoxidase deficiency.

4. **Treatment** with **penicillin, vancomycin,** or **trimethoprim-sulfamethoxazole** can decrease duration and frequency of recurrent infections.

IV. HEMOSTASIS AND COAGULATION DISORDERS

   A. Thrombocytopenia   *(quantitative platelet dysfunction)*

   1. Thrombocytopenia is the **most common cause of abnormal bleeding.**

   2. **Bleeding time** is prolonged when platelet count is $<100 \times 10^9/L$; **petechiae and purpura** may occur when the platelet count is 20 to $50 \times 10^9/L$, and **risk of severe hemorrhage** increases if platelet count is $<20 \times 10^9/L$.

   3. **Bleeding** occurs at superficial sites, for example, skin, mucous membranes, and genitourinary and GI tracts.

   4. Thrombocytopenia is **caused by impaired platelet production, abnormal platelet pooling,** or **increased peripheral destruction.**
   a. **Increased peripheral destruction**
      (1) Increased peripheral destruction is the **most common cause of thrombocytopenia** and may be immune-mediated (or idiopathic) or due to thrombocytopenic purpura (discussed next), sepsis, platelet transfusions, or certain drugs (e.g., quinidine).
      (2) **Idiopathic thrombocytopenic purpura (ITP)**
         (a) **General characteristics**
            (i) **No exogenous cause for platelet destruction** is found in the patient's history.
            (ii) **Acute form** is associated with viral infection in children and resolves spontaneously.
            (iii) **Adult form** is chronic, does not resolve spontaneously, and may be associated with other autoimmune diseases.
            (iv) Patients develop **mucosal bullae and purpura,** with mucocutaneous bleeding.
         (b) **Laboratory findings**
            (i) **Peripheral smear** reveals thrombocytopenia with large platelets; other cell lines are normal.
            (ii) **Bone marrow aspiration/biopsy** reveals increased megakaryocytes.

        (iii) **Platelet-associated immunoglobulin** G indicates immune-mediated disease.

    (c) Treatment

        (i) Patients should **avoid drugs that act as platelet antagonists** (e.g., aspirin).

        (ii) **Corticosteroids** are recommended for severe thrombocytopenia.

        (iii) **Transfusions** are reserved only for patients who have severe bleeding, because **survival time of transfused platelets** is short.

        (iv) **Plasmapheresis** is generally not effective.

        (v) **Cyclophosphamide** or **azathioprine** may be necessary for refractory ITP.

  b. Abnormal platelet pooling

    (1) General characteristics

      (a) Abnormal platelet pooling is **most commonly due to splenic sequestration.**

      (b) **Splenomegaly** (often due to cirrhosis with portal hypertension) leads to **increased platelet sequestration.**

    (2) Laboratory findings

      (a) **Thrombocytopenia in a patient with hypersplenism** suggests the diagnosis.

      (b) **Bone marrow aspiration/biopsy** reveals an adequate number of marrow megakaryocytes.

    (3) Treatment

      (a) Usually, **no treatment** is required because the degree of thrombocytopenia is not severe.

      (b) **Platelet transfusion** is of little value because the transfused platelets will also be sequestered.

      (c) **Splenectomy** may be of benefit, especially if splenic enlargement causes discomfort.

  c. Impaired platelet production

    (1) General characteristics

      (a) **Impaired platelet production** commonly occurs secondary to administration of certain drugs (e.g., ethanol, thiazide diuretics, chemotherapy).

      (b) The condition is also **associated with vitamin B_{12} and folate deficiency or may be secondary to bone marrow disease** (e.g., myelofibrosis or bone marrow aplasia), therefore affecting other cell lines.

    (2) Laboratory findings

      (a) **Bone marrow biopsy** is necessary if no obvious drug or vitamin deficiency is present that reveals bone marrow disease.

      (b) Thrombocytopenia is evident on **peripheral smear.**

    (3) Treatment

      (a) Patients should **discontinue offending agent** or **receive treatment for the underlying disease.**

      (b) **Platelet transfusion** is indicated if bleeding is present.

      (c) **Vitamin B_{12}** and/or **folate supplementation** is indicated if required.

B. Platelet dysfunction   *(qualitative)*

  1. General characteristics

    a. Platelet dysfunction is **most commonly caused by certain drugs** [e.g., acetylsalicylic acid and other nonsteroidal anti-inflammatory drugs (NSAIDs)]. *aspirin*

b. This condition is **also seen in uremia** and is therefore **not uncommon in chronic renal failure.**

2. Laboratory findings
  a. **Peripheral smear** is normal (normal number of platelets).
  b. **Platelet function study results** are abnormal.

3. Treatment
  a. The **offending agent** should be **discontinued.**
  b. **Dialysis** may benefit patients who have uremia.

C. **Platelet consumption syndromes**

  1. **Thrombotic thrombocytopenic purpura (TTP)**
    a. **General characteristics**
      (1) **TTP usually affects young women.**
      (2) **A viral prodrome** is common.
      (3) **Presence of hyaline thrombi** in arterioles without vessel wall inflammation (i.e., not a vasculitis) → microvascular disease.
      (4) **Extensive activation of the coagulation system** does not occur.
    b. **Clinical features** include a pentad of symptoms and signs: thrombocytopenia, microangiopathic hemolytic anemia, neurologic abnormalities, renal dysfunction, and fever.
    c. **Laboratory findings**
      (1) **Peripheral smear** reveals severe thrombocytopenia, schistocytes, fragmented RBCs (due to hemolysis), and increased reticulocytes.
      (2) **Coombs' test** is negative (the hemolysis is not immune-related).
      (3) **Signs of intravascular hemolysis** are present, including elevated serum LDH and bilirubin levels, hemoglobinemia, and hemoglobinuria.
      (4) **Gingival biopsy** may reveal diagnostic histopathologic changes characteristic of the disease.
    d. **Treatment** involves **exchange transfusion or plasmapheresis coupled with fresh frozen plasma;** this therapy has improved outcome.

  2. **Hemolytic uremic syndrome (HUS)**
    a. HUS is **similar to TTP.**
    b. HUS **occurs in children.**
    c. Because this disease is localized to the kidney, **no neurologic abnormalities** occur; otherwise, HUS has the **same clinical picture** as **TTP.**

  3. **Disseminated intravascular coagulation**
    a. **General characteristics**
      (1) In DIC, an **activated coagulation system leads to abnormal formation of excessive thrombin within the circulation** → consumption of coagulation factors and platelet, with activation of the fibrinolytic system.
      (2) DIC occurs **secondary to other conditions** (e.g., amniotic fluid emboli, meningococcemia, sepsis, metastatic malignancy, trauma).
    b. **Clinical features**
      (1) Clinical features **depend on balance between intravascular coagulation and fibrinolysis.**
      (2) **Extensive skin and mucous membrane bleeding and shock** occur if coagulation predominates.
      (3) Less frequently, **thrombosis** predominates, which leads to extensive clotting and peripheral acrocyanosis.
    c. **Laboratory findings**
      (1) **Peripheral smear** reveals thrombocytopenia, schistocytes, and fragmented red blood cells consistent with intravascular traumatic hemolysis.

Table 9-4
Diagnostic Summary of Bleeding Parameters

Platelet Count	Bleeding Time	PTT	PT	Likely Diagnosis
Decreased	Increased	Normal	Normal	Thrombocytopenia
Normal	Increased	Normal	Normal	Thrombocytopathia
Normal	Normal	Increased	Normal	Hemophilia A
Normal	Increased	Increased	Normal	VWD
Normal	Normal	Increased	Increased	Liver disease, lack of vitamin K, heparin therapy

PT = prothrombin time; PTT = partial thromboplastin time; VWD = von Willebrand's disease.

(2) Prothrombin (PT), **partial thromboplastin (PTT)**, and **bleeding times** are prolonged (Table 9-4).

(3) **Serum analysis** indicates decreased fibrinogen levels, elevated fibrin degradation products, and decreased clotting factors.

d. Treatment

(1) The **primary cause** should be reversed if possible, for example, antibiotics for sepsis.

(2) **Fresh frozen plasma** to replace clotting factors and **platelet** to correct thrombocytopenia are indicated in patients who have excessive bleeding.

(3) Patients in whom thrombosis predominates need **prompt anticoagulation therapy with intravenous heparin.**

D. Hereditary coagulopathies

1. Hemophilia A

a. General characteristics

(1) Hemophilia A is the **most common hereditary coagulopathy.**

(2) The disease is **X-linked recessive.**

(3) In hemophilia A, VIII^{pro} (the procoagulant portion of the factor VIII molecule) is **deficient,** whereas VIII^{ag} (the antigenic portion of the factor VIII molecule) is present in **normal amounts.**

b. Clinical features

(1) Patients have a **positive family history.**

(2) Patients are **usually men,** because the disease is X-linked recessive.

(3) **Bleeding** occurs into soft tissues, muscles, and weight-bearing joints.

(4) Bleeding occurs hours or days after injury and may persist for days to weeks, which may lead to **compartment syndromes.**

(5) **Hematuria** may also occur.

c. Laboratory findings

(1) Bleeding parameters; **PTT** is prolonged (reflects function of the intrinsic coagulation pathway), **PT** is normal (reflects function of extrinsic and common pathways), and **bleeding times** are normal (reflects platelet function).

(2) Levels of VIII^{pro} are **decreased,** and VIII^{ag} levels are **normal.**

d. Treatment

(1) Patients should **avoid platelet-inhibiting drugs** (e.g., NSAIDS).

(2) **Factor VIII concentrates or cryoprecipitates** are effective in treating bleeding and should be given **before any surgical or dental procedure.**

2. von Willebrand's disease
    a. General characteristics
        (1) This disease is **autosomal dominant** with variable penetrance.
        (2) Both VIII^{pro} and VIII^{ag} **levels** are decreased.
        (3) Because VIII^{ag} is necessary for **normal platelet aggregation, lack of VIII^{ag}** causes signs and symptoms similar to those conditions with **defective platelet function.**
    b. Clinical features
        (1) Both **males and females** are affected.
        (2) Patients have a **mixed bleeding picture,** with both mucocutaneous bleeding and soft-tissue bleeding with hemarthrosis.
    c. Laboratory findings
        (1) **PTT and bleeding time** are prolonged; **PT** is normal.
        (2) **Serum VIII^{ag} and VIII^{pro} levels** are decreased.
    d. **Treatment** involves **cryoprecipitate therapy,** as factor VIII concentrates are rich in VIII^{pro} but poor in VIII^{ag}.

E. Acquired coagulopathies
    a. General characteristics
        (1) Acquired coagulopathies usually involve **multiple coagulation factor deficiencies.**
        (2) The common deficiencies are the **vitamin K–dependent factor deficiencies.**
        (3) Other causes include **DIC** (see IV C 3), presence of **lupus inhibitor,** and **antifactor VIII antibody–mediated coagulopathy.**
    b. **Vitamin K–dependent factor deficiencies**
        (1) General characteristics
            (a) Vitamin K acts as a **cofactor in the final step of the synthesis of factors II, VII, IX, and X by the liver.**
            (b) This **deficiency** can occur **secondary to liver failure; malabsorption of vitamin K** (as with biliary obstruction that impairs absorption of fat-soluble vitamins A, D, E, and K); **malnutrition** (common in intensive care unit patients); and the **use of certain drugs** (sodium warfarin).
        (2) Clinical features
            (a) Features of the **primary disorder** typically predominate.
            (b) **Soft-tissue bleeding with hemarthrosis** may occur if deficiencies are severe.
        (3) Laboratory findings
            (a) **PT and PTT** are prolonged; **bleeding time** is normal.
            (b) **Evidence of liver disease** may be present (e.g., elevated liver enzyme levels).
            (c) **Serum levels** of vitamin K and factors II, VII, IX, and X are decreased.
        (4) Treatment
            (a) The **underlying cause** must be treated.
            (b) A dose of **10 mg of parenteral vitamin K** restores production of clotting factors within 8 to 10 hours.
            (c) **Severe hemorrhage** can be treated with fresh frozen plasma.

10

Infectious Diseases

I. CENTRAL NERVOUS SYSTEM (CNS) INFECTIONS

A. Meningitis

1. General characteristics

   a. Meningitis may be **bacterial** (Table 10-1) or **aseptic** (viral).

   b. **Most cases** occur in **children** or **young adults.**

2. Clinical features

   a. **Signs and symptoms** include fever, headache, stiff neck, lethargy, and irritability.

   b. **Palpable purpura** suggests *Neisseria meningitidis.*

   c. **Focal neurologic findings and seizures** may occur in **bacterial meningitis** but are less common in viral infections of the meninges.

3. Laboratory findings

   a. **Gram's stain of cerebrospinal fluid (CSF)** is often positive in bacterial infection.

   b. **Lumbar puncture** should not be performed if suspicion of an intracranial space-occupying lesion exists.

   c. **CSF, blood, and purpuric fluid culture studies** should be performed (Table 10-2).

4. Treatment

   a. Treatment for **bacterial meningitis** includes **intravenous penicillin G** for **pneumococcal or meningococcal disease.**

   b. **Cefotaxime** or **ceftriaxone** is indicated for patients who have *Haemophilus influenzae* infection.

   c. **Broad-spectrum antibiotics** such as penicillin and a third-generation cephalosporin should be administered until the organism is identified.

   d. **Prophylaxis with rifampin** should be administered to household contacts (younger than age 4) of patients who have ***H. influenzae*** infection.

   e. **Rifampin** should be administered to all household contacts of patients who have **meningococcemia.**

   f. **Viral meningitis** is usually self-limited and requires no treatment.

Table 10-1
Bacterial Causes of Meningitis According to Age

Organism	Group Affected
Haemophilus influenzae	Infants
Neisseria meningitidis	Adolescents and young adults
Streptococcus pneumoniae	Older adults
Listeria monocytogenes	Immunosuppressed and elderly

B. Encephalitis

    1. General characteristics

        a. Encephalitis is **usually caused by a virus.**

        b. For example, **herpes simplex virus (HSV)** may cause encephalitis.

    2. Clinical features

        a. **Signs and symptoms** include fever, headache, behavioral changes, delirium, and speech difficulty.

        b. **Seizures** may occur.

        c. A **prodrome** of upper respiratory tract signs and symptoms may occur.

    3. Laboratory findings

        a. **CSF analysis** reveals a moderately elevated protein level and lymphocytic pleocytosis.

        b. **Electroencephalogram** shows a characteristic pattern in HSV infection.

        c. **Serum analysis** that measures antibody titers to various encephalitic viruses can be helpful.

        d. **Computed tomography (CT) scan** and **magnetic resonance imaging** can reveal focal abnormalities after a few days of infection.

    4. Treatment

        a. **Acyclovir** is commonly used to treat HSV encephalitis.

        b. **Other viral causes** are treated supportively.

C. Intracranial abscess

    1. General characteristics

        a. Intracranial abscesses usually arise from **infection of a contiguous site** (e.g., ear or sinus infection).

        b. Infection is **commonly caused by streptococci** and/or **anaerobes.**

    2. Clinical features

        a. **Signs and symptoms** include fever with worsening headache, decreased level of consciousness, and vomiting.

Table 10-2
CNS Findings in Meningitis

	Bacterial	Aseptic
Cells	1000–10,000/μl	10–2000/μl
% Neutrophils	>50%	>50%
Glucose	<40 mg/dl	Normal
Protein	>150 mg/dl	<100 mg/dl

      b. **Focal neurologic signs** are present.

      c. Seizures occur.

  3. Laboratory findings

      a. **CT scan** is an important diagnostic tool because **lumbar puncture** is **contraindicated** in these patients (Figure 10-1) due to the **risk of herniation.**

      b. **Serum analysis** reveals leukocytosis; **blood culture** may be positive if septicemia has occurred.

  4. **Treatment** includes **surgical drainage** with appropriate **antibiotics** (e.g., penicillin).

II. HEAD AND NECK INFECTIONS

  A. Otitis

    1. Otitis is an **infection** that may occur **in the inner, middle,** or **outer ear.**

    2. Patients who have **outer ear infections** demonstrate minor irritation in the external auditory canal and are **treated with a topical antibiotic** (gentamicin drops).

    3. **Middle ear infections** typically occur **in children; signs and symptoms** include **ear pain** and **decreased hearing.**

      a. **Otoscopy** reveals hyperemic, bulging tympanic membrane with pus behind it.

      b. Middle ear infections are **often caused by pneumococcus,** *Streptococcus pyogenes,* or *H. influenzae;* these infections **often respond to amoxicillin** or **trimethoprim-sulfamethoxazole** (TMP-SMX).

    4. **Inner ear infections** are usually viral and are thus often untreatable; **signs and symptoms** include tinnitus and vertigo.

  B. Sinusitis

    1. **Sinusitis** is usually caused by pneumococcus or *H. influenzae.*

    2. Clinical features

      a. Patients often have a **prodrome of upper respiratory tract signs and symptoms.**

      b. **Signs and symptoms** of sinusitis include pain and stuffiness in the affected sinuses and tenderness to palpation over the affected sinuses.

    3. **Laboratory findings** are usually unnecessary for diagnosis, although **sinus radiography** may reveal opacification of the affected sinus.

    4. **Treatment** of patients who have **minor infection** includes the use of decongestants and an appropriate antibiotic (e.g., penicillin).

III. RESPIRATORY TRACT INFECTIONS

  A. Upper respiratory tract infections (URTIs)

    1. These infections are also known as the **common cold** and are usually virally induced.

    2. **Signs and symptoms** include cough, coryza, rhinorrhea with or without a sore throat, and a slight fever.

    3. **Treatment** is symptomatic because infection is self-limited.

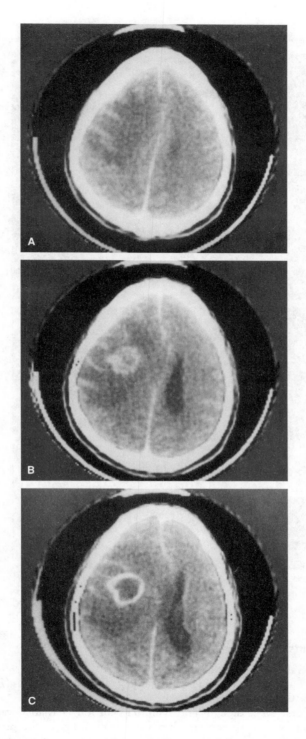

Figure 10-1. Computed tomography scan of a patient who has an intracranial abscess. Note the surrounding edema and mass effect.

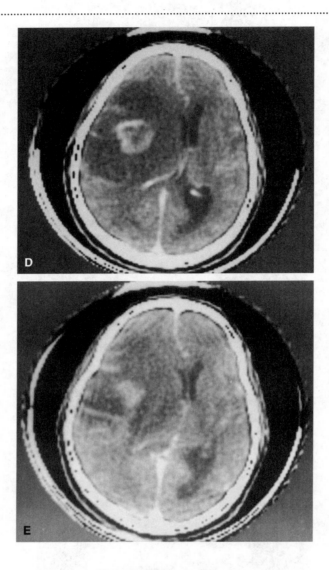

Figure 10-1. *(continued)*

B. Pharyngitis

    1. General characteristics

        a. Pharyngitis is **caused by viruses** [e.g., Epstein-Barr virus (EBV)]; **mycoplasma;** or **Group A streptococci.**

        b. Persistence of signs and symptoms for longer than 1 week, respiratory stridor, excess secretions, difficulty swallowing, or the **presence of a palpable mass** should alert the clinician to a more serious cause, such as **malignancy** or **epiglottitis.**

    2. Clinical features

        a. The **main symptom** is a sore throat.

    b. **Exudate** may be present in either a bacterial or viral infection.

    c. The presence of **URTI-like symptoms** suggests a viral pharyngitis.

    d. Malaise, fever, generalized lymphadenopathy, and splenomegaly associated with hypertrophied tonsils with a white exudate strongly suggest EBV (infectious mononucleosis).

    e. **EBV infection** is **more common in the young adult** population.

3. Laboratory findings

    a. Because clinical distinction of streptococcal pharyngitis from viral pharyngitis is difficult, a **throat swab and culture** for group A streptococcus are recommended for patients who have pharyngitis.

    b. **Monospot test results** for heterophile antibodies are positive in patients who have EBV infection.

4. Treatment

    a. **Penicillin therapy for streptococci infections** should last for at least 10 days to prevent rheumatic fever.

    b. **Viral pharyngitis** is usually self-limited.

    c. **Tetracycline** or **erythromycin** is indicated **for mycoplasma.**

C. Pneumonia

1. Pneumonias can be **community-acquired** or **hospital-acquired.**

2. Community-acquired pneumonias

    a. **General characteristics**

        (1) The **most common cause** of community-acquired pneumonia is ***Streptococcus pneumoniae*** (also called pneumococcus).

        (2) **Atypical form** is ***associated with Mycoplasma pneumoniae,*** which has a different clinical presentation from that of ***S. pneumoniae.***

        (3) Infection with **M.** *pneumoniae* is commonly seen in **young adults.**

        (4) **Aspiration pneumonia** is associated with anaerobic infections.

    b. **Clinical features**

        (1) **Signs and symptoms** include fever, chills, and a productive cough with rust-colored sputum.

        (2) If the **pneumonia** is **caused by M.** *pneumoniae,* **the cough** is **typically dry** and **hacking.**

        (3) In **aspiration pneumonia,** the **sputum** is **foul-smelling.**

        (4) **Breath sounds** are decreased over the infiltrated area.

        (5) **Pleural rub** may be appreciated.

        (6) **Splinting on inspiration** may occur.

        (7) **Signs and symptoms** associated with M. *pneumoniae* tend to be less severe.

        (8) A **history of loss of consciousness** (e.g., passing out after an alcohol binge); **seizures;** or **vocal cord paralysis** should alert the clinician to the **diagnosis** of **an aspiration pneumonia.**

    c. **Laboratory findings**

        (1) **Sputum microscopy with Gram's stain** often provides the diagnosis, revealing large numbers of neutrophils and streptococci.

        (2) **Sputum culture** confirms the diagnosis.

        (3) **Mycoplasma sputum analysis** is often less diagnostic.

        (4) **Bronchial washings** may be required if sputum cultures are not diagnostic and the patient's condition deteriorates despite empiric antibiotic therapy.

        (5) **Chest radiographs** may reveal infiltrates that are often arranged in a

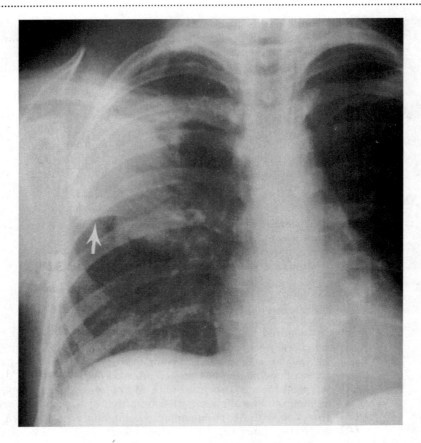

Figure 10-2. Chest radiograph of a patient who has a right upper lobe infiltrate that may be consistent with pneumonia caused by S. *pneumoniae*.(Reprinted with permission from Freundlich IM, Bragg DG: A *Radiologic Approach to Diseases of the Chest*, 2nd ed. Baltimore, Williams & Wilkins, 1996, p 246.)

reticulonodular pattern in S. *pneumoniae* and mycoplasma infection (Figure 10-2).

(6) Cavitating lesions are common in aspiration pneumonia (Figure 10-3).

  d. Treatment

    (1) **Streptococcus infections** are treated with **penicillin** either parenterally (if the disease is severe) or orally.

    (2) **Mycoplasma pneumonia** is treated with **erythromycin.**

    (3) **Aspiration pneumonia** is treated with high doses of **penicillin** or **clindamycin.**

3. Hospital-acquired pneumonias

  a. These pneumonias often involve **gram-negative bacilli** (e.g., *Klebsiella* and *Escherichia coli*).

  b. **Clinical features** are as previously described.

  c. **Diagnosis** may require bronchoscopy and lung biopsy to identify the agent.

  d. **Treatment** involves a penicillinase-resistant penicillin or cephalosporin plus an aminoglycoside (e.g., gentamicin).

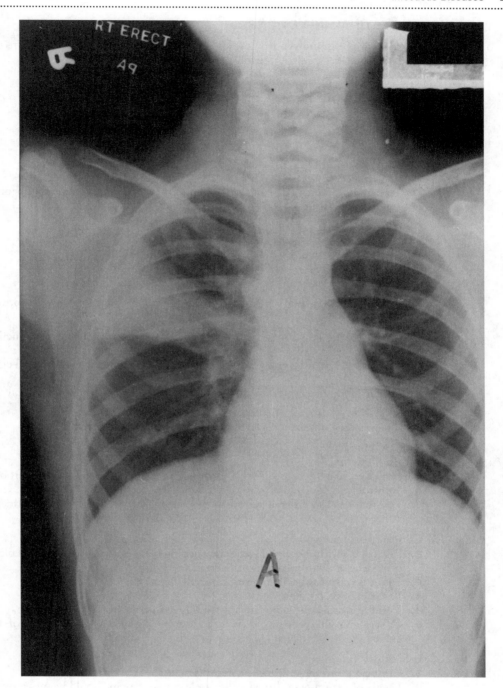

Figure 10-3.   Chest radiograph illustrating right upper lobe pneumonia (anterior segment) with multiple areas of necrosis and cavitation associated with an aspiration pneumonia. Note the horizontal fissure in the middle of the right lung field, which defines an upper lobe pneumonia.

IV. GASTROINTESTINAL INFECTIONS

A. **Diarrhea, food poisoning syndromes,** and **liver and biliary tract infections** are discussed in Chapter 6, "Gastrointestinal Disorders."

B. **Appendicitis** is also discussed in Chapter 6, "Gastrointestinal Disorders."

V. GENITAL AND SEXUALLY TRANSMITTED INFECTIOUS DISEASES

A. Urethritis

    1. General characteristics

        a. This infection occurs in **sexually active individuals** (usually males).

        b. **Urethritis** is classified as **gonococcal** (*Neisseria gonorrhoeae*) or **nongonococcal** (usually *Chlamydia*).

        c. **Infections** with both organisms may be present in a single patient.

    2. Clinical features

        a. **Dysuria** is the main symptom.

        b. **Purulent discharge** is often present in gonococcal disease.

        c. **Cloudy discharge** may be present in nongonococcal disease.

    3. **Laboratory findings** from microscopy and culture of urethral swab are **diagnostic.**

    4. Treatment

        a. **Gonococcal disease** is treated with **penicillin** or **spectinomycin** (if penicillin resistance is likely).

        b. **Tetracycline** may be given for 7 days after penicillin if chlamydial co-infection is suspected.

        c. **Tetracycline** or **erythromycin** is effective treatment for nongonococcal disease.

B. Pelvic inflammatory disease (PID)

    1. General characteristics

        a. PID is defined as infection of the uterus and other adnexal structures.

        b. **Infection** may be caused by *N. gonorrhoeae*, *Chlamydia*, or pelvic anaerobes.

        c. **Intrauterine device** use increases risk of PID.

        d. PID may lead to **infertility** or **ectopic pregnancy** due to scarring of adnexal structures.

    2. Clinical features

        a. PID occurs with **increased frequency during menses,** because menstrual blood provides a growth medium for bacteria.

        b. Patients have **lower abdominal pain.**

        c. **Fever** may be present.

        d. **Cervix, uterus,** and **adnexae** are **tender,** with **pain during intercourse.**

        e. **Cervical discharge** may be observed during **speculum examination of the pelvis.**

    3. Laboratory findings

        a. **Cervical swab** for culture is often **diagnostic.**

        b. **Levels of serum beta–human chorionic gonadotropin** should be measured to rule out ectopic pregnancy.

        c. **Appendicitis** should be **ruled out by an abdominal ultrasound.**

        d. **Pelvic ultrasound** may be necessary if a **mass** is **palpated** during pelvic examination (e.g., abscess) or if **discomfort** is so **severe** it precludes a thorough examination.

4. Treatment

a. For severe disease, the **patient** should be **hospitalized,** and **parenteral antibiotics** should be administered.

b. **Clindamycin plus gentamicin** are **often effective** when **anaerobes** are suspected.

c. **Doxycycline plus cefoxitin** is often the first line of treatment because this drug combination is effective **against both chlamydial and gonorrheal infections.**

C. Genital ulcer and lymphadenopathy syndromes

1. General characteristics

a. These conditions are **more common in males than in females.**

b. **Genital herpes** is the **most common cause** of genital ulcer disease in the **United States,** followed by **syphilis.**

c. **Less common causes** include lymphogranuloma venereum, chancroid, and granuloma inguinale.

d. **Gonorrhea** does not cause genital ulcers.

2. Clinical features

a. Features of **genital herpes** include:

(1) Onset occurs with **soreness and itching,** followed by **genital erythema.**

(2) **Herpetic vesicles** then develop.

(3) Sores eventually heal; however, **outbreaks continue** to occur throughout the patient's lifetime.

b. Features of **syphilis** include:

(1) Patients who have **primary syphilis** are initially seen with a **painless ulcer.**

(2) The **base of the ulcer** is often hard.

c. Features of **lymphogranuloma venereum** include:

(1) **Large inguinal lymph nodes** accompany the genital ulcer.

(2) This condition is **caused by** *Chlamydia trachomatis.*

d. Features of **chancroid** include:

(1) Patients have **multiple, painful ulcers.**

(2) The **edges** of the ulcers are often **undermined and rough.**

(3) **Suppurative inguinal nodes** may be present.

e. Features of **granuloma inguinale** include:

(1) Patient has a **painless lesion** with a **beefy red appearance.**

(2) The **ulcer edges** are **rolled.**

(3) **Adenopathy** is not a predominant finding.

(4) **Causative organism** is *Calymmatobacterium granulomatis;* this organism causes a slowly advancing infection.

3. Laboratory findings

a. For herpes, the **Tzanck test and culture** are **diagnostic.**

b. **For syphilis, dark-field examination and rapid plasma reagin (RPR) testing** are **diagnostic.**

c. **For lymphogranuloma venereum, culture of expressed pus** and **serologic testing for** presence of **anti–C.** *trachomatis* antibodies are **diagnostic.**

d. **For chancroid, culture of** *Haemophilus ducreyi* from the ulcer or suppurative nodes is **diagnostic.**

e. **For granuloma inguinale, scrapings of** the **ulcer edge** show Donovan's bodies with Giemsa or Wright's stain.

4. Treatment

a. **Herpes symptoms** are **self-limited but recur; acyclovir** can reduce the severity of outbreaks but is not curative.

Tidid (ticlopidine)

    b. Syphilis is treated with penicillin.

    c. Lymphogranuloma venereum is treated with tetracycline or erythromycin.

    d. Chancroid is treated with erythromycin, ceftriaxone, or TMP-SMX.

    e. Granuloma inguinale is treated with tetracycline or TMP-SMX.

VI. URINARY TRACT INFECTIONS (UTIs)

A. General characteristics

1. UTI may occur as a result of inoculation during instrumentation or sexual intercourse.

2. UTIs are **more common in females,** especially those who have vaginal or periurethral colonization.

3. Risk factors include obstruction (leading to urinary stasis) and reflux, pregnancy, diabetes mellitus, and immunodeficiency states.

4. If untreated, a UTI may lead to pyelonephritis.

B. Clinical features

1. Signs and symptoms include urinary frequency and urgency, dysuria (burning), suprapubic pain, and malodorous and/or cloudy urine.

2. Signs and symptoms of pyelonephritis include flank pain with fever in conjunction with signs and symptoms of UTI.

3. Mental status changes in the elderly may be the only presenting sign of a UTI.

C. Laboratory findings

1. Urinalysis may reveal bacteria on microscopy.

    a. Leukocyturia may be present.

    b. Positive test results for leukocyte esterase and/or nitrites suggest the diagnosis.

2. Urine culture gives definitive diagnosis.

    a. A **clean-catch midstream specimen** is required.

    b. Colonization of $>10^5$ colonies/ml is diagnostic.

    c. If the **colony count** is $<10^5$ colonies/ml, **treatment** may still be warranted if the patient is symptomatic or is known to have recurrent UTIs.

    d. If routine cultures are negative and the patient remains symptomatic, **cultures for *Ureaplasma* or *Chlamydia*** should be specifically ordered.

3. Intravenous urography may be necessary in patients who are suspected of having vesicoureteral reflux, obstruction, or renal calculi.

D. Treatment

1. Uncomplicated lower UTI often responds to TMP-SMX during a treatment course of 5 to 7 days.

2. Prolonged antibiotic coverage may be required for recurrent or chronic UTIs (e.g., nitrofurantoin).

3. Acute pyelonephritis requires broad-spectrum antibiotic coverage such as ampicillin and gentamicin.

4. Urologist referral is necessary for patients who have **anatomic obstructions,** because **chronic reflux** can lead to **renal failure.**

VII. OSTEOMYELITIS AND JOINT INFECTIONS

A. Osteomyelitis

1. General characteristics

  a. **Infection of the bone** may occur from infection at a contiguous site (history of trauma or surgery to the affected area) or from hematogenous spread.

  b. *Staphylococcus aureus* is the **most common cause of osteomyelitis.**

  c. *S. aureus* and *E. coli* infections are also **common among intravenous (IV) drug abusers.**

  d. Osteomyelitis commonly affects long bones and vertebral bodies.

  e. **Individuals with prosthetic joint replacements** have an **increased incidence of joint infections.**

2. Clinical features

  a. **Local pain** and **tenderness** may be present.

  b. **Redness overlying the infection** may be present.

  c. **Fever** may or may not be present.

  d. **Draining sinus tracts** result from chronic infections or implants.

3. Laboratory findings

  a. **Diagnosis is confirmed** with isolation of *S. aureus* from the blood and/or bone in a patient who has symptoms of focal bone involvement.

  b. If blood cultures are negative, **bone biopsy and culture** should be considered to isolate the organism.

  c. **Bone scan** is effective in localizing the site of infection.

  d. **Radiographs** are **often normal early** in the course of the infection, **because radiographic changes often lag** behind clinical onset by **as much as a week.**

  e. **CT scan** is more sensitive than plain radiographs and can localize abscesses.

4. Treatment

  a. Osteomyelitis is treated with **nafcillin or oxacillin IV for 24 weeks,** followed by an oral regimen with an antibiotic such as dicloxacillin.

  b. **Total antibiotic therapy** should continue for **4 to 6 weeks.**

  c. **Vancomycin** can be used for **patients** who are **allergic to penicillin.**

B. Joint Infections

1. General characteristics

  a. **Patients who receive intra-articular corticosteroids** and **patients who have existing joint disease** (e.g., rheumatoid arthritis) are at **risk for joint infections.**

  b. The **most common causes** are *N. gonorrhoeae*, streptococci, and *S. aureus.*

  c. *Pseudomonas* is a **common cause of joint infection in IV drug abusers.**

  d. *S. epidermidis* is a **common pathogen in individuals who have prosthetic joints.**

2. Clinical features

  a. Patients have **acute onset of monoarticular pain** that **commonly involves the knee.**

  b. **Signs and symptoms** include joint pain, swelling, redness, and decreased range of motion.

  c. Patients who have a **joint prosthesis** may **experience pain** and **loosening of the prosthesis.**

  d. **Disseminated gonococcal infection** is suggested by additional tenosynovitis and vesicopustular skin rash.

  e. **Gout or pseudogout** must also be considered in the differential diagnosis.

Idiopathic hypertrophic subaortic stenosis, the ECG tracing show
IHSS (1) *LVH* (2) *W-P-W syndrome* (3) *abnormal Q wave*

194 Chapter 10

> **3.** Laboratory findings
>
>> **a.** Joint fluid should be **aspirated for Gram's stain and culture.**
>> **b.** **Crystal disease** can be **ruled out with** a specimen for **polarizing microscopy** (see Chapter 1, "Rheumatic Diseases").
>> **c.** In **gonococcal infection, skin lesions** and **joint cultures** may be negative; however, a **cervical culture** may reveal the diagnosis.
>
> **4.** Treatment
>
>> **a.** Treatment involves **repeated aspiration of infected joint material** or **surgical drainage.**
>> **b.** **Systemic antibiotic therapy** is recommended for at least **4 to 6 weeks** if a staphylococcal infection is present (e.g., vancomycin).
>> **c.** **Gonococcal arthritis** responds well to **penicillin** within 7 to 10 days.

VIII. OTHER INFECTIOUS SYNDROMES

> **A.** Infectious mononucleosis
>
>> **1.** General characteristics
>>
>>> **a.** Infectious mononucleosis is **caused by EBV.**
>>> **b.** This disease tends to occur in **adolescence and young adulthood.**
>>
>> **2.** Clinical features
>>
>>> **a.** Patients have a **fever** and discrete, nonsuppurative, slightly painful **enlarged lymph nodes** that often involve the posterior cervical chain.
>>> **b.** **Splenomegaly** is present in approximately half of the patients.
>>> **c.** **Sore throat, anorexia,** and **malaise** are often present.
>>> **d.** **Ampicillin** may induce a petechial rash in these patients.
>>> **e.** **Exudative pharyngitis** may be present on physical examination.
>>> **f.** Occasionally, patients may develop **hepatitis.**
>>
>> **3.** Laboratory findings
>>
>>> **a.** **Complete blood count** shows an initial granulocytopenia, followed by a lymphocytic leukocytosis (leukocytes are large in appearance).
>>> **b.** **Positive Monospot test results** indicate presence of heterophile antibodies.
>>> **c.** **False-positive Venereal Disease Research Laboratory** and **RPR test results** can occur with this disease.
>>> **d.** If the CNS is involved, the CSF will show **increased levels of lymphocytes and protein.**
>>> **e.** Levels of liver enzymes and bilirubin are often elevated.
>>
>> **4.** Treatment
>>
>>> **a.** **No specific treatment** is available.
>>> **b.** **Nonsteroidal anti-inflammatory drugs** may provide symptomatic relief.
>>> **c.** **Contact sports** should be **avoided** in patients who have splenomegaly to decrease the incidence of splenic rupture.
>
> **B.** Tuberculosis (TB)
>
>> **1.** General characteristics
>>
>>> **a.** **Increased incidence** is largely caused by human immunodeficiency virus (HIV) infection.
>>> **b.** TB is **common in immigrant and underprivileged groups.**
>>
>> **2.** Clinical features
>>
>>> **a.** **Pulmonary-related TB signs and symptoms** include increased cough, weight loss, hemoptysis, and fatigue.
>>> **b.** **Extrapulmonary signs and symptoms** affect kidneys, bones, and meninges.

3. Laboratory findings
   a. **Tuberculin skin test results** are positive but indicate only prior exposure: this does not confirm that the patient's current signs and symptoms are caused by tuberculosis.
   b. **Pulmonary tuberculosis** is detected with acid-fast stain and appropriate culture of sputum.
   c. **Bronchial washings** may be necessary to obtain an appropriate specimen.

4. Treatment
   a. **Isoniazid and rifampin** are first-line therapies and should be administered for at least 6 months.
   b. **Chemoprophylaxis with isoniazid alone for the following high-risk individuals** is necessary:
      (1) Younger than 30 years of age with positive tuberculin skin test
      (2) Individuals of any age with a recently converted skin test
      (3) Individuals with a positive skin test who receive chronic steroid therapy
      (4) Individuals who are in close contact with an infectious patient

C. Eosinophilia-associated infections

   1. General characteristics
      a. Eosinophilia is **associated with multicellular parasitic infections** (e.g., schistosomes, pinworms).
      b. **Parasitic causes** must be **differentiated from allergic causes** of eosinophilia, which are commonly associated with drug reactions.

   2. Clinical features of pinworm infection
      a. Pinworms **commonly affect young children.**
      b. **Cecum and adjacent bowel** are **often inhabited** by the organism.
      c. Eggs are **laid at the anus** after infection occurs.
      d. Patients have **perianal pruritis, irritability, restlessness, and enuresis.**
      e. Patients have **vague abdominal complaints,** particularly in the right lower quadrant.

   3. Laboratory findings
      a. The **presence of eggs on perianal skin** is diagnostic.
      b. **Stool examination** may reveal adult worms.
      c. **Eosinophilia** may be present.

   4. Treatment
      a. **Oral mebendazole** is highly effective and should be used in symptomatic patients.
      b. In asymptomatic patients, **good hand-washing after defecation** and **clean bed linens** will kill the organism and prevent reinfection.

D. Toxic shock syndrome (TSS)

   1. General characteristics
      a. TSS is **caused by toxin formed by certain strains of *S. aureus.***
      b. TSS often **involves vaginal colonization by the staphylococci,** with increased incidence in females using tampons.
      c. TSS **may occur with infection at other sites** as well.

   2. Clinical features
      a. **Signs and symptoms** include fever, hypotension, desquamative rash on the hands and feet, vomiting, and diarrhea.
      b. **Nonpurulent conjunctivitis** may occur.

3. Laboratory findings
  a. **Blood cultures** are usually negative because the disease is caused by an immune reaction to the toxin.
  b. The **toxin-producing organism** may be cultured from wound scrapings or the vagina if colonization has occurred.

4. Treatment
  a. Patients require **rapid IV rehydration.**
  b. If vaginal colonization is present, the **tampon should be removed.**
  c. Antibiotics such as nafcillin are indicated.

E. Lyme disease

1. General characteristics
  a. Lyme disease is characterized by **multiorgan involvement.**
  b. The **causative organism is *Borrelia burgdorferi,*** which is **transmitted to humans by a biting tick.**

2. Clinical features
  a. Patients **initially** have a **skin rash.**
    (1) The rash **begins at the site of the tick bite** and **spreads.**
    (2) The rash is a **target-like lesion** known as **erythema chronicum migrans;** rash develops on the **thighs, buttocks, and trunk.**
  b. Patient **may develop aseptic meningitis weeks to months after the tick bite; signs and symptoms** include neck pain and stiffness, headache, and low-grade fever.
  c. **Arthritis** (usually a migratory polyarthritis) may develop months after initial infection as well.
  d. **Myocarditis** may also occur after initial infection.

3. Laboratory findings
  a. Diagnosis is established by **detection of antibodies against the organism.**
  b. **Joint fluid aspiration** for culture is negative.

4. Treatment involves tetracycline, erythromycin, or penicillin; these drugs can hasten recovery and reduce severity of late manifestations.

F. Acquired immunodeficiency syndrome (AIDS)

1. General characteristics
  a. AIDS is **caused by the HIV.**
  b. HIV is **transmitted** through sexual contact with an infected person, parenteral exposure to infected blood by transfusion or needle stick, and perinatal exposure.

2. Clinical features
  a. Individuals infected with HIV are **typically asymptomatic for years.**
  b. Signs and symptoms of AIDS begin with weight loss, fevers, and night sweats.
  c. Patients have **sinus fullness and pain on swallowing.**
  d. **Candidal oral plaques** and **gingival ulceration** occur.
  e. **Pulmonary infection** may develop and is evidenced by **increasing cough and shortness of breath.**
  f. Patients have **diarrhea.**
  g. **Difficulty in concentrating, depression,** and eventually **frank confusion** can develop.
  h. Kaposi's sarcoma, non-Hodgkin's lymphoma, primary lymphoma of the brain, and invasive cervical carcinoma occur at an increased incidence in AIDS patients.

i. **White lesions on the side of the tongue** may be noted (hairy leukoplakia).

j. **CNS involvement** may include emotional lability, psychomotor slowing, abnormalities of pursuit eye movements, and focal deficits.

3. Laboratory findings

a. **Screening by enzyme-linked immunosorbent assay (ELISA) for anti-HIV antibody** is highly sensitive; antibodies are present within several months of the infection but may not be present immediately after infection.

b. **Positive results on ELISA** should be confirmed by Western blot to detect false-positive results.

c. **Pancytopenia** is common in advanced HIV infection (it may also be a side effect of the antiretroviral therapy used).

d. **Cutaneous anergy** is common.

e. **CD4 lymphocyte count** falls as the disease progresses.

f. **Chest radiograph** may show apical infiltrates suggestive of *Pneumocystis carinii*.
  (1) **Wright-Giemsa stain of sputum** may detect the organism.
  (2) **Bronchial lavage** may be necessary for isolation of the organism.

4. Treatment

a. **No cure** exists, and the **disease is fatal.**

b. **Regular CD4 counts every 6 months** are recommended for infected individuals who have a CD4 level greater than 500 cells per μL.

c. When the **CD4 count** drops **below 500 cells per μL,** zidovudine (also known as AZT) **treatment** should be **initiated** (antiretroviral therapy).

d. **Other treatments** that show some benefit include didanosine, dideoxycytidine, and stavudine.

e. Recently, protease inhibitors such as saquinavir, nitonavir, and indinavir have been approved; use of these drugs results in reduced HIV replication.

f. TMP-SMZ is a common first-line agent for *P. carinii.*

g. *Mycobacterium avium-intracellulare* is another common infection among AIDS patients that may respond to triple antibiotic therapy (e.g., clarithromycin, clofazimine, and rifampin).

— chlamydial pneumonia — (16 wk infant)

(1) 50% has conjunctivitis

(2) lung: diffuse rales c̄ few wheezes

CXR: hyperinflation and diffuse interstitial
     or patchy infiltrates

WBC count: eosinophilia

— 10-30 minutes after ingestion of strychnine
The patient often falls into violent convulsions
Gastric lavage is postponed until treatment to prevent
the convulsions is started.